DIET IN SINUS INFECTIONS
AND COLDS

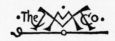

THE MACMILLAN COMPANY
NEW YORK · BOSTON · CHICAGO · DALLAS
ATLANTA · SAN FRANCISCO

MACMILLAN & CO., Limited
LONDON · BOMBAY · CALCUTTA
MELBOURNE

THE MACMILLAN COMPANY
OF CANADA, Limited
TORONTO

DIET
IN SINUS INFECTIONS
AND COLDS

By EGON V. ULLMANN, M.D.

FORMERLY SPECIAL LECTURER FOR BIOLOGY AT THE OREGON STATE
COLLEGE; INSTRUCTOR AT THE FIRST MEDICAL CLINIC AT THE
UNIVERSITY OF VIENNA, DEMONSTRATOR AT THE LARYNGOLOGICAL
CLINIC (PROF. HAJEK) AT THE UNIVERSITY OF VIENNA, ASSISTANT
PHYSICIAN AT THE OTOLARYNGOLOGICAL CLINIC (PROF. NEUMANN)
AT THE UNIVERSITY OF VIENNA, MEMBER OF THE RESEARCH STAFF
OF THE STATE SERUM INSTITUTE OF AUSTRIA

RECIPES AND MENUS
By ELZA MEZ

NEW YORK
THE MACMILLAN COMPANY
1937

PRINTED IN THE UNITED STATES OF AMERICA

Dedicated to my father

DR. KARL ULLMANN

NOTE

All proper names used in the text (with the exception of Buddha, Galen, Hippocrates, Rousseau, Koch, Virchow and Pasteur) can be found alphabetically arranged in the bibliography, page 127.

INTRODUCTION

*Optimum medicamentum est opportune cibus
datum* (Joost van Lom)

THE dietetic therapy described in this work con-
stitutes the first systematic attempt to apply the
modern knowledge of nutrition to individuals who
suffer from repeated colds and sinus diseases.

The recognition of the value of dietetics is not
new. The rules of the Monastery of Buddha, which
were written for the Monks about 2,500 years ago,
are not far from our present-day ideas of dieting.
The Monks had to sleep on hard floors. Meat, fish
and eggs were forbidden. A meal consisted of a
single dish. The first meal was taken at sunrise and
the second had to be consumed by noon. From noon
until the next sunrise no food was allowed except
water and milk. Such were the rules of dieting
2,500 years ago.

In our day such strict fasting rules are not only
unnecessary, but would certainly be harmful because
of our speedy life, full of worries and strain, which
cannot be compared with the complacent and
leisurely life of yesterday.

A great many sinus patients and people who suffer
from repeated colds are not primarily sick in the
nasal sinuses. The nasal mucous membrane simply
represents the location where abnormal reactions of

the tissues manifest themselves. In many people it represents the point of minor resistance. Much has been said about this subject, but nevertheless, no one has been able to throw any light on this somewhat confused situation. Neither the physician nor the patient can become wiser from reading any of the innumerable books on this subject. If any one had the endurance to test for himself all the advice accumulated in books, he would probably not live long enough to go through the list.

However much we may have studied, written and read about nutrition, no intelligent and systematic application has thus far been made in this direction on sinus patients. Years of experience in this line and the urging of patients and friends have brought me to the conclusion that it would be the right thing to present my experience in the form of a book. No miracle should be expected. No one should expect to find a cure-all for any disease. There will always be patients who must submit to surgery. But in directing the methods of eating and living of all the many who suffer from colds and sinus diseases, we may contribute more to the improvement of conditions than by devising a new operation. It is not the purpose of this book to change living conditions. All I hope for is that it may be a guide to the many thousands of sufferers on how to live, on how to eat, and on how to defend themselves against existing conditions.

E. V. U.

CONTENTS

DIET IN SINUS INFECTIONS
AND COLDS

I

THE PARANASAL SINUSES AND COLDS

Every other person believes he suffers from sinus trouble. Sinusitis has become a national ailment and the word, sinus, is today certainly one of the most popular medical expressions. How strange it seems that, outside of a few, no one seems to know what the sinuses really are. Beyond the fact that we can pride ourselves on having more sinus diseases than any other nation, it has naturally become fashionable to suffer from this ailment. As this book is written for all those who suffer from their sinuses, it will be best first to explain what the sinuses really are.

Every living being whom nature has provided with a voice has not only a windpipe and vocal cords, but also paranasal sinuses. The nose as a unit and organ has three functions: The sense of smell, regulation of the air we breathe, and last but not least, through the sinuses, its function as a resonance box for the voice.

Symmetrically on either side of the nose we find several cavities in the facial skull. They are arranged on three levels: on the first we find the largest, the maxillary antrum; on the second we find a number of irregular-shaped cells which are called because of their irregularity, the ethmoidal labyrinth; on the same level further back we find the sphenoid sinus; on the third level, above the orbit, the frontal sinus is located. The anatomists have divided the ethmoidal labyrinth into an anterior and posterior section. If we accept this classification, we see that on each side of the nose there are five cavities, called the paranasal sinuses, all varying in size and shape. There are no two individuals whose sinuses have the same structure; they are all different in size, shape, and the thickness of the bony walls. The walls are covered with a mucous membrane, the direct continuation of the mucous membrane of the nasal cavity. Every sinus is connected with the nasal cavity through a small opening (ostium). Unfortunately, these ostia are not only very small, but in some sinuses are located at the top of the cavity, which handicaps the outflow of accumulated fluids. To make this clear, we shall compare these cavities with a container which has an outlet at the top and not at the bottom. With the opening at the top only, the container cannot empty itself, and the bottom remains full unless it is tipped to the side of the outlet or a hole is drilled near to the bottom. This is exactly the case with some of the paranasal sinuses and explains why, in so many cases, the sinuses have to be washed out. Under normal conditions these sinuses are filled with air which forms the medium for the vibration of sound.

The paranasal sinuses form the resonance box for the voice. Just as all musical instruments consist of one part which produces the tone and another part which makes this tone sound, so it is with the human voice. The individuality of an instrument is conditioned by the shape, size and material of its resonance box. While the strings of all violins may be of the same material and the same length, the difference in violins depends on the shape and material of the body. In this alone lies the value of the violin.

If we compare the vocal cords to the strings of the violin, we can look upon the paranasal sinuses, together with the oral cavity as the resonance box of the voice. The differences in shape, size and thickness of bones are responsible for the quality of the voice. The training and education of Caruso, Patti and Jeritza was not altogether responsible for the quality of their voices; the ideal physical conditions of their throats and noses were probably more responsible for it.

Every man contracts colds, regardless of the climate in which he lives. A normal person contracts a cold usually during the change of seasons (fall or spring) and suffers from it for approximately a week. He then forms an immunity which lasts from six to eight months protecting him until the next season. At the same time a great many others in the same community suffer from colds, and science deducts, mainly from this fact, that a simple cold is a contagious disease, though no definite organism or bacterium has thus far been found which can be held responsible. Age-old observations have shown us that a sudden change of temperature, moisture in the air, and a sudden change of climate, favor the development of a cold. It is evidently due to a combination of circumstances and not to one factor alone, since as frequently happens a large group of people simultaneously suffer from colds.

In every cold the mucous membrane of the nose becomes congested. As the mucous membrane of the nose is continuous through the small ostia with the mucous membranes of the sinuses, the congestion will often narrow the ostia of the sinuses if it is severe enough, and will eventually close these sinuses from the outside, impairing their ventilation in this way. All mucous membranes contain glands, which constantly secrete. If a sinus is closed in this way the secretions will accumulate under pressure. This acts as a further stimulant to secretion and the sinuses will fill up more and more. Emptying will become more difficult as congestion increases, and we find ourselves in the midst of a vicious circle. If we consider that millions of bacteria are always present in a healthy nose, living there as saprophytic parasites, we cannot wonder that they find, under these circumstances, favorable conditions to propagate. Within a day or two pus develops and the sinuses become infected. We see, therefore, that even a common cold affects the sinuses. In the majority of cases, however, the congestion of the mucous membrane during a common cold will diminish on the third or fourth day, thus not lasting long enough to close the sinus openings entirely but clearing up soon enough to establish proper ventilation again, which will counteract the propagation of germs and lead to recovery.

Not all sinuses necessarily become infected during a cold. Very often we see that one side or even one sinus only becomes infected. This depends largely on the anatomical condition of the particular nose, as all noses vary considerably in this respect. Cases of unilocular sinus infection will, as a rule, need some kind of surgical intervention, thereafter healing and not bothering the patient any more.

What has so far been described, takes place during a common cold. Nevertheless, a large number of people contract not only one cold a year, but are subject to frequent colds and are unable to overcome them for a long period of time. It is only natural to expect that in all of these cases the sinuses become infected. In exactly these cases we find frequent complaints of rheumatism, arthritis, neuritis, vague headaches, fatigue and constipation—in other words, complaints which definitely indicate to the thinking observer that something is fundamentally wrong with the organism. The concept of focal infection which has developed within the last fifteen to twenty years has predominated medical thinking, in some instances to the exclusion of age-old experiences, and has led to the belief that the bacteria always found in those infected sinuses are the cause not only of the sinus disease itself, but also of the many accompanying ailments.

We have neither clinical nor experimental proofs that sinus diseases are infectious or contagious. For quite a while this concept predominated as a consequence of the bacteriological era of Koch and Pasteur. We should rather look for a fundamental change in the organism, which makes our system more susceptible to the development of colds and all their consequences. Lacking a clearer definition, this condition is called *lowered resistance* or a *run-down condition*.

Having observed these conditions for many years, I tried to find constitutional symptoms which are common to all these patients. I found that in all cases of colds and sinus infections the patients showed symptoms of a marked acidosis. One can observe that patients during these conditions become short of breath very easily and if examined for this show that they are unable to hold their breath after a deep inspiration longer than 20 to 25 seconds while the normal individual is able to retain his for an average of 40 seconds. This, however, naturally varies as to the degree of acidosis. With the increase of acidosis the length of time for which a deep breath can be retained will diminish.

The depth of breathing is regulated by the concentration of carbonic acid in the blood which acts as a stimulant on the respiratory center in the brain. The carbonic acid is formed as a waste product during the process of oxidation in the organism. Increased oxidation means, therefore, increased acidity. Thus with increased acidity the breathing becomes faster and shallower and more carbon dioxide is released through the hyperventilation. The time a deep breath can be retained by an individual is therefore a fairly good, although a rough estimate for the degree of acidosis. We recognize here a mechanism of the organism for the regulation of the blood reaction.

Another far more reliable and exact method of determining the degree of acidity is the examination of the hydrogene-ion concentration of the urine, a procedure to be described later.

In directing the method of living and eating of these patients so that this acid condition is counteracted, their resistance can be built up and in most instances they will be kept free from colds.

Many of my patients have been free from colds for two years since I put them on a proper diet, while, prior to that, they had from four to six colds during each winter.

In the literature of the past three years, a few scattered reports appeared about the influence of diet on sinus diseases. In some of these reports (Jarvis, Glasscheib) the important rôle of acidosis was emphasized. But no systematic and persistent effort has so far been made to stress the *necessity* of dieting in these diseases, and the few reports published to date have not received the attention they deserve.

In order to avoid confusion, it should be made clear now that what is said in this book cannot be applied unconditionally to allergic diseases. There are a great many people suffering from hay fever and asthma whose sinuses are diseased. Hay fever and asthma are frequently caused by external sources; that is to say, pollens, dusts, etc. These will not be included in our problem.

II

GENERAL ADVICE TO PEOPLE SUFFERING FROM COLDS

Food alone will not bring about a cure if not aided by general hygiene. It may at first sound paradoxical to say that the more civilized we live the more favorable are the conditions for contracting colds. Nevertheless it is true.

Every one knows that our rooms are overheated, but no one seems to want the heat lowered. The maximum temperature for rooms we sit and work in quietly should be 68 degrees. The fact that it is cold outside during the winter does not necessitate the raising of the temperature indoors. For the same reason we should not overheat our rooms on a cool summer day. The custom of lighting the fireplace of comparatively small rooms in an already heated house, especially during spring and summer, is detrimental. It is different in an hotel lobby or in a very large living-room. The keeping up with the "Joneses" is a temptation for people who live under entirely different circumstances to do as the "Joneses" do.

Mr. and Mrs. Smith have company. They live in an average modern apartment house where the indoor temperature is kept around 70 degrees. If five or six people sit for a few hours in their living-room, the temperature will automatically rise from 70 to 73 degrees. In order to make this room more cozy, the hostess lights the fireplace. This brings the temperature well up to about 78 or 80 degrees. The women feel quite warm but the men very uncomfortable. Every one is perspiring. Now is the time to serve iced drinks. After spending four or five hours under such conditions they go out into the cold night. Is it any wonder that two days later somebody of this party has a cold?

No one doubts the merits, advantages and comforts of our bathing facilities, but people who are inclined to colds should not bathe daily. The loss of epithelium during this process will make them more sensitive to the differences in temperature, especially after hot baths. If we add the possibility that the temperature of the bathroom is not kept at the same degree as that of the rest of the house, a few minutes of exposure with a wet skin may be responsible for a fresh cold.

Swimming is a source of catarrh and colds in many of our school children. If children were raised from early childhood with the idea of hardening them, if they were left out of doors a great deal, if they slept on an open porch and went barefooted on the lawn for a couple of hours every day and were exposed regularly to the morning sun in a bathing suit, they would be hardened enough to the change of temperature so that they would not contract colds even if they went swimming in winter. It is naturally different with all those who have been or are suffering from sinus diseases, particularly after a sinus operation. They should refrain from swimming until the physician finds it safe for them to swim again. Diving, especially, will have a bad effect on these persons because the water, which often contains irritant agents such as chlorine, will be forced into the nasal sinuses.

The same benefits, or even more, can be gained from a sun bath as from swimming. For plants, animals and man, the sun is just as important as food. The sun preserves life, keeps our cheeks red and makes the pale and sallow skin like velvet, giving it a natural brownish tint. Such a skin reacts much better and more promptly to the stimulant of warmth and cold and provides through its reflexes, a healthy blood circulation. Unfortunately, it is not always possible for civilized people to take sun and air baths regularly, but we certainly should remember them during our vacation time. For the daily routine, twenty minutes of morning exercises before an open window should be done regularly. Weak and convalescent persons should go back to bed for a short time after these exercises. They should for the first few days exercise only by rubbing and massaging the legs and arms. Later they may proceed to regular gymnastics.

A sun bath causes profuse perspiration and an increased blood circulation on the surface of the body. It increases our metabolism. An exposure to the sun for an hour may be followed by a reduction of weight, often as much as a pound. The sweat evaporates very rapidly in the sun, produces accelerated consumption of heat and stimulates the heat regulation of the body. The most efficient rays of the sun are the ultra red and the ultra violet. Unfortunately, much of their effect is neutralized through the glass of our windows. Fumes, fog and smoke decrease the effect of the sun rays in the city territories. The full effect of sun treatment may therefore be expected only in elevated districts with pure air. Too much exposure will cause a burn, for which reason one should begin to expose gradually, say from five to ten minutes at a time, and distribute the sun rays over the various parts of the body. The earlier in the morning the sun bath is taken the milder will be the reaction on the skin. In large cities, and during the winter when we cannot take sun baths, a well-planned and well-conducted treatment with sun lamps or ultra-violet lamps will be very beneficial. In children with sinus diseases, the diet, together with a systematic sunlight treatment (artificial or natural), will always lead to the best obtainable results.

The skin is a sense organ which informs us of atmospheric changes. People whose skin is weakened and relaxed are unnaturally sensitive to the most minute change of temperature. They lack the normal vigor of the skin, and due to their poor heat regulation, perspire very easily, become distressed by the least draft and are subject to frequent colds. They imagine that they suffer from rheumatism, which is far from the truth. What they really suffer from is the lack of normal skin reflexes.

Every living thing needs motion. For man, walking is the most natural, but the automobile and the paved road have made walking difficult and even dangerous. Golf, fishing, tennis and many other sports can hardly replace a regular and comfortable walk. The danger with all these various sports is that of trying to out-do the others. Although it is healthful to exercise long enough to become tired, it is unwise to become exhausted. The tiring after exercising corresponds with the feeling of saturation after eating.

It is unnecessary to stress to the American public the importance of cleanliness.

A word may be said here about constipation. Refined foods cause and favor constipation, and constipation favors and causes acidosis. Instead of taking laxatives one needs only to eat coarser food with plenty of butter and olive oil, and better results will be obtained. The diet I advise may be followed in the beginning by some constipation, especially in cases where bread has to be restricted. In these cases it will be better to use a mild enema with Camomile tea for a few times until the bowels have adjusted themselves to the change of food. It is of especial importance to watch for constipation in all cases that are inclined to have headache.

Children have to be treated with particular care, but give even better results than adults if the diet is properly applied. Impaired nasal breathing must be surgically corrected, but surgery does not seem to help in chronic sinus diseases of children. If allergic factors as hay fever, for instance, can be excluded, the diet should always be applied. These children often suffer from lack of appetite, which makes it difficult for them to eat a whole meal. I therefore stress the importance of feeding small amounts of food frequently instead of three full meals a day. This will be discussed more fully later.

Advising a patient to keep to a certain diet without first knowing his circumstances, occupation and individual characteristics can never lead to complete success. It must be kept in mind that this, as well as other dietetic treatments, can never be sold wholesale and should always be adapted to the individual. Only the principles can be given here.

III

FOOD AND CIVILIZATION

LABORATORIES and investigators all over the world have spent their energies to find what we should and must eat if we want to avoid deficiency diseases and acidosis. Nowadays every one knows that if food lacks certain ingredients, which science calls vitamins, certain diseases will develop depending on which one of these vitamins is absent. These established facts no one can doubt. They have stood the test in thousands of animal experiments. We know a certain number of vitamins, A, B, C, D, E, and a definite number of diseases which stand in relation to them. Thus far nature has been kind enough to unveil the secrecy of her mystery. All attempts, however, to treat people affected with so-called lower-resistance and those subject to colds with any of the known vitamins has shown very little, if any, results. The problem is far more complicated.

We are inclined to generalize the results of our experiments and often create a style rather than a scientific method. This has happened innumerable times in the progress of mankind, and it is particularly noticeable in the medical field. When the pendulum starts to swing, it very often swings too far. The concept and treatment of sinus diseases

and colds within the last fifty years was dominated
at first by our achievements in anatomy and clinic.
Consequently, it developed into a specialty. Then
surgery came into the field, and prevailed even more
since the teaching of focal infection, which urged the
use of surgery, gained recognition. Many disap-
pointed patients are responsible for the large number of physicians who have turned their hopes to the
teaching of vitamins. None of these concepts alone,
however, has led us farther in accomplishing a cure.
But eventually, all of them together may attain this
goal.

Let us consider for a moment the way the American people of today eat and live. A report on diets
in the Proceedings of the Mayo Clinic (Barborka)
of August, 1931, states that "the American diet contains a large proportion of concentrated foods low in
vitamins, residue and alkaline minerals, and high in
carbohydrates and acid minerals. Such a diet lacking certain protective foods, a term applied to milk,
eggs and fresh leafy vegetables, conduces to an early
advent of degenerative diseases. Not only is this
true, but diet each day bears evidence of its imme-
diate influence on the emotions and nature of individuals." The term "deficiency disease" has been
applied primarily to the results obtained from feeding animals food lacking in one or more vitamins.
Similar results of vitamin deficiency have been
observed in man and are called scurvy, rickets, pellagra and beriberi. Very few of these diseases, however, are observed in the United States. The term
"deficiency disease" should be used on a larger basis,

including conditions in which one or more of the other nutrient substances, such as carbohydrates, proteins, fats, or minerals, may be lacking. The influence of food deficiency is just beginning to be appreciated. More and more diseases are being seen unassociated with a symptom complex which would allow their classification as a definite malady. We know definitely that scurvy is due to the lack of vitamin C and rickets to the lack of vitamin D; that is to say, we have thus far discovered the cause of diseases due to the lack of only *one* vitamin. All that is necessary in order to cure scurvy is to give the patient lemon or orange juice; to cure rickets, cod-liver oil. But what if conditions exist in which none of the known vitamins *alone* are effective but the remedy may lie only in the concerted action of many circumstances of an unknown nature? Therein, as we shall see, lies the secret of our lowered resistance.

This can be understood best from an historical viewpoint. Not simply a few thousand, but millions of years, have to be considered. We must start with the time when man emerged from the animal world and began to live his own life. His faculties, which enabled him to adapt himself more and more to the conditions of his environment, helped him to be victorious in the struggle for existence. Our physique is adapted to these conditions far beyond our comprehension. Light and warmth, air and water, plants and animals, have influenced our organism. The adaptations and characteristics we acquired in this struggle for existence are all suitable for the preservation of life, and whatever nature once created she preserves obstinately and secures by deep-rooted faculties—the instincts.

The life of animals, as well as our own life, is secured by instincts. Together with intelligence and judgment we were able to free ourselves from our environments and subdue the powers of nature to our needs. Even today we can admire the safeness of instincts in primitive people. But as soon as man was able—thanks to his intelligence—to transform nature and his environment by technical means, he reached the zone of danger in which the self-regulating security of the instincts was no more sufficient. Not only did man become exposed to danger while deviating from the natural way, but the domestic animals and plants which he cultivated around his settlements suffered also. For the wild animal only one natural way of feeding is possible. The question of survival is principally a quantitative one. The security of survival is limited to the quantity of food. This is different with domestic animals. No wild animal would take artificially changed food, as for instance does the dog or the hog. We, therefore, cannot observe diseases among the wild animals such as we see daily among domestic animals. Losing the integrity of the instinct for taking food means, therefore, a constant danger to health.

In ancient times we already meet indulgence in food and refinement in nutrition. Hippocrates and Galen have recognized the danger of this indulgence. The students of history have often pointed out how much indulgence and over-refinement in eating have contributed to the decline of the Roman Empire.

In the Middle Ages eating habits were very simple, even among the high social classes. With the discovery of new continents and new territories a new era of prosperity started and the population, especially in the cities, began to over-indulge in food and drink. But this was still limited to a rather small group of people and as the technical supplies at that time were very modest, the fundamentals of nutrition remained unchanged. Therefore we see at that time the detriment of malnutrition limited to small groups who were less malfed than underfed. The dietetic traditions of ancient times were still alive well toward the end of the eighteenth century. They prescribed very rational, and often surprisingly correct ways of how to behave and how to eat during acute diseases with fever, during injuries and various maladies.

These traditions practically fell into oblivion at the beginning of the nineteenth century. This corresponds with the time when natural sciences and technique started to transform the Old as well as the New World in its social and economic foundations.

Cities started to grow and to absorb the rural population to such a degree that, while the country population of an hundred years ago just about held its own up to our days, the population of the cities increased from between seven to fifteen times. With the expansion of the cities, more and more rural territory was absorbed and the industrial suburbs and boroughs had to adapt the same methods of living as the cities themselves. Methods of living mean, first of all, methods of eating. The accumulation of masses within a small territory interrupted the intimate connection between the individual who cultivates, and the soil which produces the living food. The people were deprived of the free choice of food and became dependent on mediators, commerce and industry, technique and transportation.

Still our grandfathers did not need to walk longer than ten or fifteen minutes from the city center in order to reach cultivated ground. Every family had a garden and kept up an intercourse with the neighboring villages, which allowed it to cover its daily needs in products of the soil, such as milk, vegetables and fruits. The poorer people were still in most cases able to gather herbs and fruits from the near-by lawns and forests—oraches, watercress, stinging nettles, dandelions and many others whose names cannot even be remembered by our parents. Many vegetables were preserved by the housewife in harmless and simple ways. Only a very few spices and colonial products were bought as they were rather expensive. Today we are compelled to buy everything. Self-provision gave way to foreign-provision; near-provision was replaced by far-provision and mass-provision and, worst of all, the free choice of food was replaced by compulsory food which the capitalist and industrialist chose to be good enough for us if they could but see a profit in it for them.

A diet developed accordingly. The concentrated foods came to the foreground as their value increased with the distance necessary for transportation. Meat, fat, sugar, cheese, cereals were in greatest demand and all the fresh vegetable foods which required more space and could not be preserved over a long period of time had to step back. We can recognize here the same economic reasons which make it more lucrative in a country with prohibition to bootleg concentrated brandy than light wine and beer.

Technique proceeded—we call it progress. It provided us with methods of preserving even vegetabilic food and gave us canned food. There is no objection against canned food in its place, for our civilization practically compels us to make use of it. But it should replace only such foods as we cannot get in a fresh state because of climate, season, or location. It is most deplorable that industry and capital were successful, by shrewd advertising methods and even with the aid of medical schools, in making people believe that canned food can replace fresh food at any time and in any way. This is far from the truth. Whatever the scientific departments of the canneries may emphasize and advertise, it is clear that the food which has been processed, heated, sugared, pickled, stained, bleached, seasoned with salt and various acids and finally closed up in a tin can, is far from its natural state. It may still contain the vitamins A, B, or C, but it never will be the same as fresh food. Especially is this true as far as acids are concerned. Whenever food is closed up in a metal container it is merely a matter of time until certain acids form. The United States Bureau of Chemistry, recognizing this fact, has twice made

the attempt to obtain a new legislation which would
compel the labeling of cans with an expiration date,
just as vaccines and sera have to be labeled.* Both
times the canneries and their allies were able to
suppress these efforts. It may be remembered by
every one that the use of canned food should be
restricted to the absolute minimum in spite of all
the advertising. Especially should one be careful
of buying canned food at sales. All these bar-
gains are the remains of one year or more and the
risk of bad effects stands in no relation to the
saving. If we are to believe the advertisers, we
must come to the conclusion that there are only
first-class products on the market in every field because everything is advertised as the best. Advertising is primarily a means toward making more
money as every businessman knows. Here, however, we are not concerned with the merits of advertising but only with preserving health and prevent-
ing colds.

Similar conditions prevail with grain products.
Innumerable books have been written, and nothing
new, I am afraid, can be said about white flour.
Authorities, such as Plimmer of London, McCollum
of Baltimore, Ragnar Berg of Germany, and many
others have devoted part of their lives to this question. But it seems to be a fight against windmills
to stop the course of time. The flour the average
American eats daily in every piece of bread, bun,
biscuit, cruller, cracker, cake, pudding, pie, waffle,

* Report of Dr. Tom at the fiftieth annual meeting of the New
Jersey Sanitary Association in Atlantic City, December 6, 1924.

and wafer is notoriously decalcified, demineralized and therewith devitalized. Not only that, but in order to appeal to the eye of the consumer who lives under the illusion that the whiter the flour the purer it is, the flour is bleached by chemical methods whose principles rest on extracting the color with a strong acid, either nitrous acid, aluminum sulphate, or chlorine gas. At the time we eat it all that remains of the grain as it grows is pure starch, which has turned acid by the chemical processes while all the ingredients which make up the vitality are extracted. To make things worse, baking powder has been invented as a convenience for the housewife. While in previous times yeast, a vitamin in itself full of wholesome minerals, was added to the bread to make it rise, we now use baking powder—one more addition to deaden the food.

Civilization first did all that it could to devitalize our food and now is making spasmodic efforts to find the vitamins (life-giving ingredients), which it first eliminated. We should not need any of these artificial aids if we could feed our population with food in its natural state. There are a large number of diseases connected with nutrition. One could even say that the wrong food given with an abundance of vitamins will lead to chronic diseases. We know from animal experiments that mice can be fed for a long time on fresh milk alone without damage. But if we feed the component parts of milk individually, as casein, butter, lactose and minerals the animals do not survive. We see, therefore, that whole and unprocessed food must be given as nature provides it if we want to survive. Galenus has said:

"Sanus homo nullum cibi genus fugure debet quo populus vivit." (He who wants to remain healthy shall avoid no food on which common people live.)

If one looks over the tremendous number of animal experiments which have been made in laboratories all over the world, one would be inclined to believe that man is in need of large amounts of vitamins. I am firmly convinced that this is exaggerated. The life of man in prehistoric times really proved that life can be preserved with only a little food. The important thing is that this food be fresh and neither broken up, bleached, refined or processed. If the organism is supplied with a variety of food in its natural state, it will not suffer from deficiency diseases.

A large, if not the largest, amount of food in our diet is taken in an unnatural state, meaning that the food is altered in some way. Food as it grows does not only consist of chemically pure proteins, sugars, fats, minerals and vitamins but is an organic compound of these various constituents. Therein lies the main value of its content of energy. Rubner found that the energy, which the animal body takes from the food, is subject to the laws of energy in nature. By heating and processing food we lose not only essential ingredients but also energy. Bircher-Benner expressed the same thought by saying that only food which contains the *living energy of the sun* retains its full value. Calories alone will not do, nor will vitamins and minerals alone; only the organic combination will provide for the full *sunlight-energy* of the food.

The historical point of view was necessary for the

better understanding of how we arrived at our present-day eating and the habits which followed. It is natural that with the change of time our ideas and theories underwent a change. The old physicians treated more or less empirically and thought that all life rested within the body fluids. In order to change these fluids, which they blamed for all diseases, they resorted to diets to a great extent which they thought would change the body fluids from acid to alkaline, from thinner to thicker, from little to more or vice versa. This old concept of humoral pathology prevailed from olden times up to the middle of the eighteenth century, the dawn of the technical age. With the invention of the microscope, the cells were discovered and every disease was blamed on them. The doctrine of cellular pathology dominated in medicine for more than forty years. Simultaneously with Virchow's cellular pathology, Koch and Pasteur introduced their discoveries of bacteria and started the bacteriological era, which still dominates today. In its exaggerations it has brought about conditions which justify the saying that we are more concerned about the weals and ills of the bacteria than we are about the diseased body. Since the war the study of chemistry is coming more and more into the foreground within the medical profession, and with it, more attention is being paid again to the body fluids. The old humoral pathology is now becoming modern again and we, therefore, are recognizing the value of diets to a greater extent than ever before in history.

IV

INFLUENCE OF THE VARIOUS FOODS

SOMETHING is wrong with the way we eat. Not every one is conscious of it and not every one likes to believe it, nevertheless it is the truth and cannot be denied by any one who has eyes to see and ears to hear. If nothing else can prove this truth, the fact that the largest laboratories and the best brains of all civilized nations are indefatigably working on this problem, can. The question is not only what is wrong and how we can prove it, but what is the measure for this right or wrong.

Only the needs of the body can give the answer. To recognize these needs is a much more difficult problem than it seems to be at first. The effects of wrong nutrition may very easily escape recognition. Here the cause and the effect are not so evident as in an accident or an infection. In an acute poisoning, we recognize the effect of the poison within a definite and limited time and know what nature will do. In a case of malnutrition, we have to deal with a summation of small repeated damages. R. Berg says that "the body consumes the damaging factors slowly, buries them in its depths so that it is impossible to recognize them. After years or decades only does the transformation of the system become evident to the extent that it manifests itself as a disease." This may happen so late that the disturbance of the health can no more be recognized as the consequences of malnutrition.

In the last analysis, we must recognize these conditions as a disturbance of the original balance in the composition of the food in our nutrition. McCollum, to whom we are indebted for many new facts and their interpretation concerning nutrition, says, "An experiment within the human nutrition extending over nations has been carried out with a diet which no people in history ever tried to live on. The effects of such an experiment could in no way be predicted because we were ignorant of the dietetic qualities of the various foods and knew but little of the body needs. After an experience of two generations with a diet, consisting of white bread, meat, sugar and comparatively little potato and with an addition of small amounts of other food insufficient to balance the inadequacy of the main constituents, it has been possible to prove that certain detrimental effects were due to an improper diet." In another place he says, "One of the principal factors which brought the civilized man into a condition of physical inferiority compared with his barbaric ancestors, is the character of his food."

In our problem concerning the disposition of people who are inclined to colds and diseases of their sinuses, we have to deal with a tendency toward *acidosis*. With this expression we do not mean a condition which has up to lately been called acidosis in the medical profession. Formerly we used this expression only in conditions where the basic-acid equilibrium of the blood was disturbed. This, however, is true only in extreme cases of starvation, diabetic coma, intoxications during pregnancy and poisoning. But here we deal with people who show a fast metabolism, burning up their reserves with a surplus of acid. If such people live on food which has a surplus of acid constituents, their constitutional disposition will be aggravated instead of counter-balanced. Nearly all patients who are inclined to frequent colds are of a rather nervous type. They are often restless, easily worried and often cannot control their temper. A husky, phlegmatic, calm patient with a chronic sinus suppuration is always an exception. If, therefore, anything could be expected from dietetic measures, they must be directed in such a way that they will counteract this fundamental disposition.

In order to understand the principles of the diet it may be well first to study the influence of various foods and how they are best used for our purpose.

V

PROTEINS

At the time when the studies of systematic nutrition began, more attention was given to the proteins than to any of the other foods. The principal reason was that proteins are very high in caloric value and therefore seemed to be the most important of all foods.

The formula of Voit was followed for more than half a century prescribing for a man of seventy kilograms, who did average work, 120 gm protein, 55 gm fat and 500 gm carbohydrates, equal to approximately 3,000 calories per day. These figures were regarded as correct by most physiologists until the time of the World War. The disturbed possibilities of providing enough and proper food for whole nations started a new era of research. All eyes were opened to the fact that not only were these figures not absolute ones, but one began to doubt even their relative value. Not until the United States Bureau of Health came out with the report, after years of experimental research, that the protein needs lie from 70 down to 25 gm for 70 kilogram of body weight per day, was general attention called to this important fact. Further research has shown that the more accurate the examination the lower the figure of our protein needs. All examinations leading in this direction are based upon the experiments of Chittenden who, some twenty-five years ago, began cautiously an experiment on himself to see how low he could reduce the protein in his diet and not interfere with his well-being. To his surprise he remained in nitrogen equilibrium and in an improved physical condition on a diet which contained no more than 36.72 gm of digestible protein. Chittenden felt so convinced that this reduction of the intake in proteins resulted in a marked improvement in his physiological well-being that he determined to test this problem on a larger scale. This led to his well-known and often quoted experiments with a group of faculty members and a volunteer group of Yale students. This experiment showed that the very students who proved to be the best athletes had lived during the nine months of the experiment on a diet which was the lowest in protein content as compared with the diet of the other participants. The figures of Chittenden were so surprising that they attracted the attention of research men in all countries, with the result that the experiment has become the foundation of modern protein nutrition.

The best and most minute examinations made it very probable that the protein content of 20-30 gm per day is sufficient for our well-being if the relation of minerals, vitamins and non-proteins to the proteins is correctly chosen. It has to be considered that the normal loss of proteins in an adult person is approximately 25 gm per day. Theoretically our daily food should be sufficient to cover this loss, but unfortunately we do not yet know which one of the food-proteins is best to cover the needs of the body. It is for this reason that we have to advise a larger amount of proteins than the minimum amount of 25 gm per day, if we want to avoid mistakes and malnutrition.

The latest research allows the conclusion that an amount of 70-80 gm total protein will cover the daily needs and avoid malnutrition. With this latter amount the body is provided with one-half to two times more proteins than are actually needed. That is done as a safety factor.

The largest amount of proteins in our food are represented by meat, but the fact that one can live on vegetarian food alone has been proved so often that no one has the right to doubt it. Is meat then indispensable? Since olden times people, nations and religious sects have abstained from all meat, chiefly because they did not believe in killing animals. About the middle of the nineteenth century, the vegetarian movement began. The name "vegetarian" does not derive from vegetable, but comes from the latin word *vegetus*, meaning healthy, full of strength. The most frequent form of vegetarian diet is the lacto-vegetarian, one which accepts food of the living animal, such as milk and eggs. If the old vegetarian movement was not successful in its time, it was because the evaluation of the various proteins was still unknown. We naturally can cover the needs for fat and carbohydrates with vegetables, but the needs for proteins out of vegetabilic food can be covered only if such a diet is carried out very scientifically. A proof that this was evidently not

done is shown by the cartoons of half-starved vegetarians in the papers of that time, which probably
still can be remembered by older people.

The whole question of an exclusive vegetarian
diet rests upon the problem of proteins. The old
vegetarian had to consume huge amounts of bread
and legumes, viz., beans, peas and lentils, in order
to cover the needs for proteins. Today we know that
the proteins contained in grain and legumes are in-
complete proteins and cannot compare in vital value
with other proteins. These old vegetarians therefore
did not provide their organisms with proteins sufficient to keep them well. Modern physiology and
modern science of nutrition have shown that we can
provide enough proteins with vegetable food if we
eat enough green leafy vegetables, potatoes, nuts
and soy beans. If we consider that this type of food
has a rather large surplus of alkalis, and will in combination with fruits provide, besides the proteins, a
satisfactory quantity of minerals and vitamins, it
would be a non-recognition of the truth if we should
still maintain the belief that one cannot live exclusively on a vegetarian diet and remain healthy.

The majority of people still believe that about
thirty-five to sixty per cent of the needed proteins
should be covered by animal proteins (meat).
Anything said or written to prove the contrary of
this belief can only be for the improvement of
health. Considering the fact that meat is composed
mainly of high-grade proteins with some fat and a
small amount of vitamins, we have to recognize it
as a strong acid former.

We know from the research of the last fifteen

years that we can provide high-grade proteins to cover all the needs of the body entirely out of vegetable food, especially if we realize that this type of food simultaneously contains all necessary inorganic bases and vitamins. In defense of the necessity of taking meat and its importance for our well-being, one reads in most textbooks about the dietary habits of the Eskimo living on the northwest coast of Greenland. His food comes almost entirely from animals. No part of the carcass is thrown away. Contrary to the common belief that the Eskimo lives mainly on fish and sea food, Ekblaw, who lived among the Polar Eskimos, reported that fish is an insignificant part of their diet as they catch salmon only a short period of each year, and no other fish is included in their diet. It is upon the sea birds and sea animals that they depend for food. They are not satisfied with eating the meat of these animals only, but they also drink their blood and use the stomach and intestinal contents. They evidently feel instinctively the importance of the basic elements contained in the blood as well as in the stomach contents. According to late reports of Greenland explorers (T. W. Hutchison, H. Mc-Cracker), they take in addition to meat a considerable amount of vegetable food which they obtain from Iceland moss, reindeer lichen and moss roses. From these plants the Eskimo makes his blood-purifying spring soup which he consumes in large amounts. According to previous reports, the Eskimo seems to enjoy excellent health. McCollum mentions the Eskimos as a most interesting group of people because in spite of their diet, no symptoms of rickets have ever been found among them. However, we have every reason not to believe too much in the excellent health of the Eskimo, as Hindhede and others reported his sensitiveness to infectious diseases, colds, tuberculosis and scurvy during the winter.

The fertility of the Eskimo women is very low, this being the reason that the price of a girl with an illegitimate child is a higher one than that of a virgin.

Hindhede reports that the mortality of the Greenlanders at the time when they still lived exclusively on animals was between fifty to one hundred per cent higher than that of the Danish people. Since they have imported grain products, this difference went down to eleven per cent. The mortality of men all over the world has always been greater than that of women, and a great number of authorities believe that one of the reasons is that men, everywhere, are larger meat eaters than women.

In connection with this, a word may be said about the very interesting report of Kuczynski concerning his experiences with the people of the Kirgis-Dsungaric steppe. These people live exclusively on meat, milk and kumys (fermented mare's milk). As a consequence of this nutrition, the author reports their tendency toward skin diseases, tuberculosis, frequent colds, leading to ear troubles and deafness, gout, rheumatism and kidney diseases. The gerontoxon (a dimness around the cornea which normally comes with old age) could often be found in people around thirty years of age. The sexual life of these tribes was very emphasized, leading frequently to sexual neurasthenia and hysteria. These observations fully agree with those made every day amongst civilized people. Occasionally one hears of a person living in the best of health up to the age of a hundred who has lived most of his life on meat only, but no conclusions can be drawn from that. The human organism is so adaptable that in some instances it may not be impossible for singular individuals to live for years and decades on an improper diet. There are exceptions to all rules, and one should never generalize.

Contrary to the experience with people who live exclusively on meat, no definite symptoms of malnutrition could ever be found in people living on vegetable food, if full use was made of all varieties and the food was intelligently prepared.

It cannot be denied, however, that meat has certain good qualities. It provides protein in such a concentrated form that only a multiple quantity of vegetables could provide an equal amount of proteins. Therefore, one has to eat more vegetables per weight in order to get sufficient protein.

Many people claim to have no trouble digesting a steak but feel distressed after eating a full dish of vegetables. This is partly due to prejudice and partly to the preparation of the food. In spite of all the good qualities of meat, the modern science of nutrition can no longer give it the favored position among food that it held for centuries.

While we do not exclude meat entirely from our

diet, we want to have it restricted to an amount where its acid-producing factors can easily be balanced by other food.

A word about *gelatin:* It replaces other proteins to the extent of approximately sixty per cent. It differs chemically but little from the protein from which it is derived. The animal amins, tryptophan and tyrosin, are not present. Consequently, gelatin cannot be used exclusively as the protein part of a diet.

Gelatin is easily digested. One hour is needed for its complete peptonization in the stomach. It has the advantage of fixing a good deal of acid and is thus of service in cases of hyperacidity.

VI

THE IMPORTANCE OF AN ALKALINE DIET

In order fully to understand the foundation of modern nutrition and especially of the diet advised in this book, it will be best first to recall briefly the elementary teachings of chemistry that we all learned once but which most of us have forgotten.

All substances in nature consist of simple parts, the elements. These are divided into *metals* and *metalloids* (non-metals). The most important ones are:

1. *Metals:* Aluminum (Al); Barium (Ba); Bismuth (Bi); Calcium (Ca); Copper (Cu); Gold (Au); Iron (Fe); Lead (Pb); Lithium (Li); Magnesium (Mg); Manganese (Mn); Nickel (Ni); Potassium (K); Silver (Ag); Sodium (Na); Strontium (Sr); Tin (Sn); Titan (Ti); Zinc (Zn); Zirconium (Zr).

2. *Metalloids:* Arsenic (As); Boron (B); Bromin (Br); Carbon (C); Chlorine (Cl); Fluorine (F); Hydrogen (H); Iodine (I); Nitrogen (N); Oxygen (O); Phosphorus (P); Silicon (Si); Sulphur (S).

In nature these elements are rarely isolated. They are found in the form of chemical compounds. If we want to understand the laws by which these compounds are formed, we have first to make clear that all elements, as well as compounds, can be diminished by physical methods into particles beyond which further physical diminution is impossible. We call these smallest particles *molecules*. (Molecula= smallest part). By electrical or chemical means we are able to split these molecules further into *atoms* beyond which a further division is impossible.

While the elements consist of one atom only, we find in the chemical compounds several atoms combined. Furthermore, we find that one atom can bind one or several other elements. With the above-mentioned symbols, chemical science indicates one atom. If an element is represented in a compound with several atoms, the respective number is added on the lower right to the symbol. The formula for water, for instance, H_2O means that one molecule of water contains 2 atoms H=Hydrogen and 1 atom O=Oxygen. A number before the formula indicates the number of total molecules. $2H_2O$=2 molecules water. The finer methods of chemistry enable us to measure, in spite of their smallness, the magnitude and weight of the atoms. These weights are so infinitely small that they cannot be used for practical purposes. One Hydrogen atom weighs 0,000000000-00000000000083 milligrams, which is one eighty-threehundredthousandtrillionst part of a milligram. In order to express these incomprehensibly small weights for practical purposes, we express their *relation* to the atom-weight of Hydrogen. This latter is accepted as=1. The atom-weight of Oxygen is sixteen times that of Hydrogen. Gold, one of the heaviest elements, has the atom-weight of 196.7, which means that one atom of Gold is 196.7 times heavier than one atom of Hydrogen.

The chemical formulas indicate the atom-weight. H_2O means that one molecule water contains 2 atom-weights Hydrogen and 1 atom-weight Oxygen. If the atom-weights were expressed in gram we should find in the water 2 gram Hydrogen combined with 16 gram Oxygen. The sum of the atom weights in a molecule gives the *molecular-weight*. For instance, in water we find the molecular-weight 18. ($H_2O = 2 + 16$.)

After this is clear, we can proceed to two new concepts, which are important in order to understand our discussion later.

1. *The valency.* This indicates the maximum amount of atoms of Hydrogen which can be bound to an element. The element Chlorine (Cl), for instance, has the valency 1. Its combination with Hydrogen is therefore HCl (hydrochloric acid). Its combination with Sodium is NaCl (table salt). Oxygen has the valency II (formula of water=H_2O). Many elements appear with several valencies, so we find Nitrogen with a valency III and V and Carbon with a valency II and IV.

2. *The equivalent weight,* by which we mean the magnitude of weight of an element, is just enough to bind one atom of hydrogen. According to what has been said above, it is for Oxygen 8. The amount which one equivalent weight of an element expressed in gram contains, is called the equivalent of an element because it is chemically equivalent to one gram Hydrogen. These equivalents play an impor-

tant rôle in the study of nutrition. Their magnitudes, however, are so small in the food, as well as in our body, that for practical calculations one thousandth part of an equivalent was introduced, which is called *milli-equivalent*. The equivalent of one matter is naturally always equal to the equivalent of any other matter.

Chemical compounds originate in a way that all valency groups saturate each other. A free valency group can never be contained in a chemical compound.

Theoretically, figuring out a formula, one calculates with atoms and molecules as free valencies, the so-called *radicals;* for instance, Methyl CH_3 or Methylen CH_2. These formulas are merely used as a working hypothesis and never exist free in nature. They become free only during chemical reactions, but then only for immeasurably short intervals.

The most important chemical reactions which have to be considered in nutrition and physiology are:

1. Combination with Oxygen or combustion= oxydation. Carbon (C), for instance, burns into carbonic acid (CO_2).

2. *Extraction* of *Oxygen*=reduction.

3. The *formation* of *salts.*

A salt is a body which consists of two substances with opposite characteristics; an acid and an alkali. These two substances, if combined, neutralize each other and form a new body with entirely new characteristics, a salt.

With the exception of the bones, only one-fifth of

the minerals in the animal body is found in the form of true salts. Their main purpose is to take part in the chemical transformation in the body. Some of the salts are necessary for the up-keep of the osmotic pressure. The greater part of the minerals, however, is so intimately bound with organic matter that we can liberate it only after burning the latter up. After the organic substances of the body have gradually been used up and destroyed through the processes of life, these minerals burn to alkalies and acids, respectively, then combine and form the salts.

If the free salts were allowed to accumulate they would increase the osmotic pressure of the blood and body fluids to the point of danger. The mechanism of the skin, intestines and kidneys provides for their elimination.

For a long time it has been known that the minerals which the process of life burns to acids, can only be excreted in the form of salts.

Salkowski discovered this important fact in 1871. As was previously shown a certain amount of alkali can bind only a certain amount of acid according to the equivalent weight. If the reactions of life or an unbalanced nutrition produce more inorganic acids than the present inorganic bases are able to saturate, the acids will attack directly or indirectly the proteins of the body, out of which combination the base ammonia is formed. Only with its help can the surplus acids be transformed into salts. This is a defensive mechanism of the body.

It has been one of the greatest merits of modern nutrition and physiology that R. Berg was able to show that with an acid diet the protein decomposition differs greatly from the normal because outside of ammonia other nitrogen-containing residue is produced, whose appearance in the urine has to be considered as pathologic. Berg, therefore, came to his postulate: Healthy food must contain on the average more equivalent weight of inorganic bases than is necessary for the saturation of the simultaneously consumed inorganic acids.

Conforming with the old observations of Salkowski and the newer ones of McCollum, Plimmer and others, Berg's metabolic experiments have shown another highly important point. In the previous chapter, we have seen that the concept of the daily needs of protein has changed from the figures of Voit, who gave 120 gm as a daily need to a figure of around 70 gm and even less. Berg's examinations have shown that the exploitation of the protein is most advantageous and the needs of the body for protein is the least, if the body disposes of a sufficient amount of inorganic basis. This can be best achieved if the food contains at least twenty-five thousandths equivalent weights (milli-equivalents) of alkalies more than acids per day.

The alkaline diet in granting a better chemical utilization, seems not only to contribute much to the well-being but also provides possibilities to produce the same labor with less nutrition than an acid diet.

Uric acid, for instance, which plays a great rôle in metabolic diseases, develops to excess with an acid diet, while in an alkaline diet it will be found only in negligible amounts. Its elimination is greatly impaired by acid food because the acid urine cannot dissolve its salts. An alkaline urine can dissolve approximately one hundred times more uric acid than can an acid one.

In a number of diseases this theory has stood the test of practice. In diabetes, neurasthenia, migraine, and diseases which are characterized by the deposits of uric acid in the body, the alkaline diet reduces this acid to a minimum.

The laity often speaks of acid blood. We find the same concept in the older medical literature. This, however, is not true. The base-acid relation, or in modern terms, the hydrogen-ion concentration of the blood does not change. The body controls enough mechanisms to keep the reaction of the blood always alkaline. This alkaline reaction is necessary in order to neutralize the constantly developing carbonic acid. The moment the alkalinity of the blood approaches neutrality, the transport of carbonic acid to the lungs ceases and death occurs. This is the case in acute poisoning with acids or in diabetic coma.

In examining the urine of approximately 250 patients suffering from sinus suppuration and frequent colds, I found that with the exception of three, all showed a high acidity indicated by a low pH. The more acute their condition, the more acid their urine. If one examines the urine during the interval between colds, the acidity is less but the urine is still too acid. I have seen patients who showed an acidity of 4.8 to 5.1 during an acute cold, and improved during the interval to a pH of 6.6. This means that the urine was, during the time they were free from colds, still twenty-two times more acid than the blood. In chronic sinus cases a similar parallel can be drawn. The longer the duration the more acid the urine. The acidity of the urine indicates the degree of acidosis. The only reference in literature, I could find concerning these observations is the research of Mittermaier, who examined the acidity of the nasal discharge. A comparison between his examinations and mine is exceedingly interesting. The nasal secretion is the more acid, the more acute the symptoms. It is the more acid, the more purulent the discharge. In chronic cases the acidity depends on the duration of the case. The longer the duration the more acid the nasal discharge. The reaction of the secretions changes gradually toward alkalinity with recovery.

The findings in secretions of allergic cases, which seldom are purulent, were not so regular and proved in a large percentage to be alkaline. This, too, corresponds with my findings in urine examinations. Mittermaier, however, drew from his highly interesting observations no practical conclusions as to the metabolism.

In conclusion, nothing better can be said than R. Berg's statement: *"In acid-rich and alkaline-poor nutrition, the food is utilized with the formation of residues, but with diminished possibilities for the excretion of these residues. The residues cause various diseases, diminishing the full energy of the food and increasing the need for food.*

With a sufficient alkaline nutrition, on the other hand, the body makes use of the food in the best possible way, the formation of residues is decreased by a better burning, the elimination of residues is facilitated, the utilization of energy increased and the need of food diminished."

In practice, the following division can roughly be used as to the acid-basic effect of food:

Acid	Neutral	Basic
Cereals	Vegetabilic oil	Vegetables
Meat	Butter	Fruits
Fish	Sugar	Milk
Eggs	Tapioca	Potatoes (white)
Coffee		Nuts
Tea		

The next table will demonstrate the basic and acid value of the various foods calculated in milli-equivalents. These figures naturally are not absolute ones. In examining the chemical ash value of food, various factors have to be taken into consideration. The differences of external conditions in the cultivation of the food, the type of ground and fertilizer and the influence of conservation have a very important influence on the results of the chemical analysis. Although the figures in this table are correct as to the acid or basic value, the examinations of food in other laboratories and countries may vary as to the accurate figure. They, therefore, can indicate only an average value.

FOOD TABLE SHOWING ACID AND BASIC VALUES *

Contents of 100 g of	1/1000 equivalent weights (Milli-equivalents)		
	Bases +	Acids —	Sum
FATS			
Hog lard	0.69	5.12	— 4.43
Palmin	1.11	12.47	—11.36
Margarine (vegetable fat)	20.96	28.27	— 7.31
Butter	15.98	19.97	— 3.99
MEAT			
Smoked bacon	31.97	40.55	— 8.57
Pork middle fat	15.35	27.82	—12.47
Beef middle fat	12.37	49.66	—37.29
Veal	13.14	36.10	—22.96
POULTRY			
Goose meat without bones	18.00	42.50	—24.50
Chicken meat without bones	20.07	44.39	—24.32
EGGS			
Egg without shell	17.12	39.35	—22.23
One chicken egg	6.85	15.74	— 8.89
FISH			
Herring, fresh	13.90	26.60	—12.70
Herring, pickled	534.43	552.78	—18.35
Sea Pike, fresh	16.44	35.96	—19.52
BLOOD			
Beef blood	18.57	10.79	+ 7.78
Pigs blood	17.43	12.49	+ 4.94
DAIRY PRODUCTS			
Raw full milk	15.60	11.39	+ 4.21
Whipping cream	10.67	7.52	+ 3.15
Hand cheese	102.77	122.56	—19.79
Cottage cheese	12.82	30.12	—17.30

* This table is taken from R. Berg: Grundlagen einer richtigen Ernährung, 7th Ed. Dresden, 1930.

FOOD TABLE SHOWING ACID AND BASIC VALUES
(Continued)

Contents of 100 g of	1/1000 equivalent weights (Milli-equivalents)		
	Bases +	Acids —	Sum
GRAINS, BREAD, LEGUMES			
Cream of wheat	13.38	23.57	—10.19
Rice red with silver skin	23.63	57.93	—34.30
Rice polished	4.66	10.25	— 5.65
Oat, polished	23.26	33.24	— 9.98
Noodle	9.36	14.47	— 5.11
Whole rye bread	25.00	31.00	— 6.00
Finer rye bread	22.17	24.75	— 2.58
Finest white bread	11.02	17.69	— 6.67
Lentils	28.85	46.65	—17.80
Peas, yellow	35.86	39.27	— 3.41
Beans, white	45.71	50.00	— 4.29
NUTS			
Hazelnuts	24.04	24.25	— 0.21
Walnuts	12.89	20.61	— 7.72
ROOTS, BULBS			
Potatoes	15.25	7.95	+ 7.30
Carrots ...:.....................	15.64	6.10	+ 9.54
Turnips, cabbage	10.53	7.34	+ 3.19
VEGETABLES			
Peas, young green	21.87	16.72	+ 5.15
Rose kale	16.25	26.12	— 9.87
Green kale	27.63	23.63	+ 4.00
Crisp cabbage	11.94	6.79	+ 5.15
Kidney bean, French bean	17.17	7.02	+10.15
Spinach	39.32	26.23	+13.09
Red cabbage	15.83	9.54	+ 6.29
Cauliflower	11.58	8.49	+ 3.04
White cabbage	22.39	14.18	+ 8.21
Sauerkraut	?	?	?
Lambs lettuce	15.03	10.25	+ 4.78
Asparagus	9.06	7.56	+ 1.50
Lettuce	21.30	7.17	+14.12
Rhubarb stems	13.65	4.72	+ 8.93

FOOD TABLE SHOWING ACID AND BASIC VALUES
(Continued)

Contents of 100 g of	1/1000 equivalent weights (Milli-equivalents)		
	Bases +	Acids —	Sum
FRUITS			
Dates, dried	23.22	19.13	+ 4.09
Prunes, dried	35.90	20.90	+15.00
Figs, dried	42.24	14.43	+27.81
Plums	8.41	2.61	+ 5.80
Cherries	7.92	4.08	+ 3.84
Apples	3.31	2.37	+ 0.94
Prunes	8.18	4.10	+ 3.99
Pears	6.16	2.90	+ 3.26
Oranges	12.46	2.85	+ 9.61
Peaches	10.61	4.17	+ 6.44
Strawberries	6.61	4.85	+ 1.76
Gooseberries	14.13	4.68	+ 9.45
Red currants	8.90	3.00	+ 5.90
Apricots	8.65	2.11	+ 6.54
Blackberries	10.05	2.91	+ 7.14
Raspberries	9.72	4.43	+ 5.29
Huckleberries	2.74	1.31	+ 1.43
Cranberries	6.30	11.10	— 4.80
Tomatoes	20.72	7.05	+13.67
Cucumbers	70.08	38.58	+31.50
SUGAR			
Refined, white ....neutral		neutral	neutral
Brown, raw (Barbados)	89.63	29.63	+60.00

VII

BREAD

THE question of white flour bread against whole meal bread seems to be answered satisfactorily in books. In practice, however, it is not. Ninety-five per cent of the population still live on white bread, therefore, we must deal with this question in a somewhat extensive way.

A longitudinal section of a grain of wheat is seen to consist of an outer layer of bran, enclosing the relatively large kernel (endosperm) of starch and gluten, the compound protein. At the base of the grain is a tiny germ, the portion which develops into a root and two small primary leaves when the grain is planted. The bran forms fourteen per cent of the grain, the germ but two per cent and the kernel eighty-four per cent.

The kernel, which is the part used for making white flour, consists of starch and protein with some cellulose and mineral matter but no vitamins. The bran contains a great deal of cellulose, some protein, a high proportion of phosphate of potash and vitamin B. The germ contains fat, iron and vitamins B1, B2 and E, but it must be borne in mind that the germ is exceedingly small. So we may make a rough division and say that starch and protein are supplied by the inner kernel, and mineral matter and vitamins by the bran and germ.

In the earlier processes of grinding wheat in stone mills most, though not all, of the bran was removed, but the germ was left, the resulting meal or flour being known as whole meal. By the modern methods of milling, the germ and all the bran are first removed and the kernel alone is used for making flour. It is characteristic of the wheat kernel that it is richest in protein immediately under the bran envelope, the proportion of starch rising and the proportion of gluten falling toward the center of the grain. This decrease of protein toward the center is, however, very slight. On the whole, protein is fairly evenly distributed throughout the grain. By the elaborate methods of modern milling practice, it has been found possible to obtain the flour from the different layers of the kernel in separate grades. What is known as the finest flour is yielded by the central part of the kernel, which, consequently, contains most starch and least protein, and this very white substance is used for pastry and fancy breads. The remainder of the flour is divided into three grades, representing different layers of the kernel proceeding outward toward the bran. Ordinarily white bread is made from Grades 1 and 2. Grade 3 flour, which is a little richer in protein, turns somewhat dark when baked.

Two factors have operated in determining this very complete change in the preparation of wheat flour; the first is the interest of the milling industry and the second is *public demand*. Bran is exceedingly difficult to grind, but it is easily removed by a first crushing, and the modern miller finds that it pays him to get rid of it altogether. He would not trouble about the germ but the germ contains fat which becomes rancid and certain bodies which ferment; consequently, flour containing the germ will not keep. When flour was a local supply, the miller ground just sufficient grain to satisfy current demands, but the vast quantities of flour now milled in America and Canada are stored for long periods, and for this reason it is essential that the germ should be removed, which is very easily done in the mills.

That, however, is as far as the miller wished to go. The grading of flour is entirely a question of popular demand. Instead of sinking colossal sums in elaborate machinery, the millers would have preferred to grind the entire kernel with a set of plain rollers and supply a slightly brown meal at a uniform price. But the truth is that people in America generally, and particularly the working classes who do heavy manual labor, prefer soft white bread and white pastry flour. It is only the comparatively few who will eat the darker flour, the great mass of the population dislikes it intensely. The desire for white flour foods is little less than a *craving*.

It would be of the greatest importance as far as the food value of bread is concerned if the protein content could be retained or even increased. An effort in this direction has been made in recent years by using the soy bean in bread. This is especially important for countries which cannot cover their needs for wheat and have to import it. The conflicts

in the Far East between China, Japan and Russia
are partly a fight for the soy bean. Thirty per cent
of the raw material for bread produced in Manchuria
is soy beans. Russia, Italy and recently Germany
have tried to add soy bean flour to their bread. Besides its high protein content, it consists of sixteen
per cent oil. Osburn and Mendel, Sansum as well as
Rubner, emphasized the value of the soy flour as an
addition to bread flour. Due to its protein content
it raises the food value of rye bread far above that
of wheat bread. It is very easily digested and provides the consumer with a larger amount of vegetable proteins than does any of the other breads.
Rubner advises the addition of ten per cent soy
bean flour to the usual mixture of rye and wheat.
This has the effect of better balancing the carbohydrates and sugars by the protein content of the
soy flour.

If we consider the efforts the other nations have
to make in order to obtain the necessary amount of
grain for their daily bread, it is deplorable that the
people of America, who dispose of such a wealth of
grain, do not make better use of it. Especially in
America, civilization, habit and style are responsible
for the restriction to bread made almost entirely of
refined white wheat flour, which is taken either in
the form of toast or any of the various marketable
forms such as crackers, crullers, biscuits, rolls, buns,
cakes, pies, puddings, waffles and wafers. The consequences are: Lack of calcium, valuable minerals
and vitamins, a tendency toward acidosis, poor teeth
and last, but not least, complaints about gas and

constipation. I therefore advise my patients to eat rye bread, graham bread or pumpernickel whenever the condition of the digestive tract allows the use of coarse bread. Whole wheat may be used if a finer-grained bread is required. Bakers have recently developed an excellent health bread using two parts of wheat flour and one part of lima or soy bean flour, together with raisins, nuts, yeast, and other ingredients which go into the making of bread. I am in full accord with Sansum in his hope that a wide use of this new non-acid bread will be effective in both the prevention and treatment of this type of acidosis. Rice, when used, should be unpolished and cereals should be restricted to oatmeal and corn-meal.

The carbohydrates preferably used in desserts will be described in the recipes.

The difference between whole and refined cereals may best be demonstrated in the two tables opposite.

RICE

	Potassium	Sodium	Calcium	Magnesium	Iron	Phosphor	Sulphur	Chlor
Unpolished	0.67	0.21	0.15	0.41	0.07	1.56	0.08	0.03
Half polished with the silver skin	0.28	0.09	0.12	0.14	0.01	0.84	0.03	0.00
Refined without skin	0.07	0.01	0.01	0.03	0.00	0.18	0.00	0.00

The following table gives the figures for various forms of bread, showing the inferiority of refined white bread:

BREAD

	Potassium	Sodium	Calcium	Magnesium	Iron	Phosphor	Sulphur	Chlor
Coarse dark (pumpernickel)	0.53	0.48	0.06	0.08	0.01	0.37	0.38	0.48
Whole rye	0.31	0.26	0.03	0.06	0.00	0.38	0.22	0.22
Refined white	0.09	0.17	0.01	0.03	0.01	0.23	0.20	0.42

VIII

POTATO

SPECIAL attention must be given to the potato as a food standing, as it does, between pure carbohydrates and vegetables. It is one of the most valuable food stuffs we consume, and, being very cheap, is available to every one.

It contains plenty of minerals, especially potassium, and its proteins are biologically extremely important. Its content of anti-scurvy vitamin C is of particular importance during the winter months. The Danish scientist, Hindhede, proved by an experiment on himself that man can live longer than a year on potatoes and fat alone and feel well.

It must be remembered that potatoes have to be prepared correctly. This means they should be steamed unpeeled or baked in the oven. The preparation of potatoes is a good illustration of how the preparation of food can change its typical content. One can even tell by eating the potato how it was prepared.

The following tables * show the loss of fresh substances in 1,000 gm of peeled potatoes in comparison with the same amount of unpeeled potatoes after boiling:

* Reported in the doctor's thesis of Marie Voigt.

	Loss of fresh substance per 1,000 gm
Peeled potato	
Through peeling loss of 20%....	200 gm
Through watering loss of 2.62%..	10 gm
Through boiling loss of dry substance 14%	58 gm
Total	268 gm

	Loss of fresh substance per 1,000 gm
Unpeeled potato	
Through peeling after boiling 10%	100 gm
Through boiling loss of dry substance 6%	2 gm
Total	102 gm

Besides this, it is of greatest importance whether the potato is boiled; or steamed, as is illustrated in the next table. From 100 gm of fresh potatoes, the following amounts were extracted by steaming and boiling processes:

DIFFERENCES IN BOILING AND STEAMING POTATOES

		Loss of total dry substance	*Loss of minerals*
Boiling	a. Peeled	2.4 %	14.5 %
	b. Unpeeled	0.31%	1.95%
Steaming	a. Peeled	1.14%	10.95%
	b. Unpeeled	0.07%	0.64%

We see that the greatest loss occurs in the boiling of peeled potatoes and the least loss in the steaming of unpeeled potatoes. The loss would still be greater if distilled water were used as it then would increase 17% more than in the table shown above.

The potato may be used as an object of practical experiments in Home Economics schools. To demonstrate the fact that water really extracts the most valuable parts of food, a teacher should have his students do the following experiment: One girl boils peeled potates in distilled water; the second girl puts the peeled potatoes on the stove in cold water; the third does the same with boiling water; the fourth steams peeled potatoes; the fifth puts unpeeled potatoes on the stove in cold water; the sixth puts unpeeled potatoes on the stove in hot water; the seventh steams unpeeled potatoes, and the eighth bakes unpeeled potatoes in the oven.

Without knowing anything about the purpose of the experiment, the pupils will be able to tell by tasting the potatoes by which method the most minerals were left. They will express their findings by saying that one potato needs a great deal of salt, another less, and the third no salt.

For various characteristics and qualities, potatoes are very useful in every diet. In *reducing diets,* potatoes are taken as a foundation because they easily satisfy and because of their protein-saving carbohydrates. On the other hand, they have a relatively low caloric value. Furthermore, it has to be considered that with no other food of so little protein content will a N-balance result. For reducing purposes, potatoes are best used in combination with fruits.

In *constipation,* potatoes taken in an amount of 1½ pounds per day will produce voluminous, bulky moist stools.

In *kidney diseases,* potatoes are sometimes temporarily used as the main dish. This is done at times when one wants to lessen the burden of the kidneys. In this case, the potato must naturally be prepared without salt.

In *stomach diseases,* potatoes find a large field as food. Here they are used as a mush and, together with butter or sour cream, may represent the main part of the diet.

In *fattening treatments,* the potato is valuable because of its readiness to absorb fats. Two hundred grams of potato will absorb 40 gm of butter or 60 gm of thick cream without becoming unpalatable.

In *diabetes,* it is valuable for the same reason. Here it stands in preference to bread.

In all people who show a tendency toward *acidosis,* especially to the formation of uric acid (rheumatism, gout) the potato is important because of its lack of purin bodies. An abundance of consumed potatoes has a uric acid dissolvent effect.

Especially for this latter-mentioned quality, potatoes should be used freely by people who have *frequent colds.*

IX

FRUITS

MANY people not familiar with this problem may be surprised to hear that their acid condition can be corrected to a great extent if they will eat sour fruits. The taste of food is often misleading as to its biologic effect. Sour and sweet are opposite sensations of taste, but not chemical contrasts which can neutralize each other. One can speak of sweet-sour dishes. The chemical contrast to acid is basic or alkaline. Whenever an acid and an alkali combine, a salty taste results. There are three ways of evaluating the chemical action of food; first, by taste, second by the chemical ash value, and third by its biologic effect. Citrus fruits, for instance, have a highly acid taste but a marked alkaline effect in the body, while meats or bread are neutral in taste and have an acid effect. In 1914 Blatherwick demonstrated the specific influence of the ash in foods on the composition of urine. The conservation and the preparation of food, especially prolonged cooking and warming over may change alkaline into acid food. From this point of view Kroetz introduced the conception that the ash value of a food cannot be relied upon entirely to give a true picture of its metabolic result. A food's metabolic value can be determined only by what Kroetz calls its biologic effect in the human body.

We, therefore, can neglect the taste-value of food entirely as it does not indicate anything as to its biologic effect. While the ash value is the basis of all nutritional examinations, we should in practice always consider the conservation and preparation of the food together with the ash value in order to come to the only true result, the biologic effect. It is the biologic effect only which in the end will always be the main object of every therapy.

This may be the place to say a few words about vitamins. There is probably no word in the literature of nutrition which has become more popular than the word vitamin. It has previously been explained that so far we know about six or seven vitamins only. Every one of these known vitamins stands in definite relation to some disease. We emphasize the importance of vitamins A, B, C, D, E, etc., in the food although none of the diseases which are due to the lack of these vitamins have been known to be common in this country with the exception of rickets. In spite of this, we have to recognize the fact that diseases are seen which, we feel certain, are due to some deficiency in nutrition, but we do not know exactly just where to look for this deficiency. As said before, we expose ourselves to deficiency diseases by processing food. It is true that canned tomatoes contain the anti-scurvy vitamin and it is true that canned spinach contains vitamin A, but have these or any other vegetables been examined as to what has been lost by the canning process? All the scientific departments of the canneries can possibly do is to look for *known* ingredients, but the unknown ones are probably of equal importance. For a person with symptoms of malnutrition, the advice to take large doses of vitamin A, B, or C, will not help because he is neither suffering from xerophthalmia nor from pellagra, beriberi or scurvy. What he really needs cannot be defined, in so far as we have not yet unveiled nature to the extent that we dare say there are just so many vitamins and no more. But we do know from the study of vitamins that they all are contained in fresh food. We may hope to discover more vitamins, or whatever is understood by this name, in the future. As long as we do not know more, we must insist that people under suspicion of malnutrition or deficiency diseases must be fed with fresh food only, if we want to be sure that they do not miss any important ingredient of whose nature and effect we are as yet ignorant. Only to this extent am I opposed to canned food.

Many times a diet consisting exclusively of raw food has been advised with the idea of not cooking or even heating the food in order not to destroy the vitamins, minerals and other important parts. That the idea leading to such a diet is sound and has great merit cannot be denied. But a diet consisting exclusively of raw food meets with so many objections from the patient, as well as from the physician, that its application is impracticable. Through hundreds of generations man has been used to a mixed diet. The sudden change of going back to the rank of the ape as far as eating is concerned, cannot be expected to be accomplished without disturbances. A diet of exclusively raw food is so filling and at the same time so low in caloric value that it must lead to undernourishment. For the same reason it is entirely inadequate for moderate and cold climates. Last, but not least, it is not advisable from the viewpoint of public health because of its likelihood of carrying infections. However, *recognizing the merits of raw food, I recommend the juices of raw unprocessed fruits and vegetables as a means of overcoming the difficulties and disadvantages of a raw food diet.*

Various extreme food faddists have advised at different times that we live entirely on fruit. While it is like every other extreme, unnecessary and frequently harmful, we want, however, to consider a few of the good points in its favor. The considerations concern exclusively fresh and dried fruits.

Apples. The apple contains the highly valuable iron, which is so important for the blood. The fruit acids of the apple have a stimulating effect on all the excreting organs in the body. The caloric value is relatively well utilized by the body. In eating six pounds of raw unpeeled apples, only 11.7% of the caloric value is lost through the stools.

Pears. The pear is important for its high sugar and calcium content. These two are often found together in fruits. The pear tastes sweeter than the apple not because of the higher sugar content, but because of the lower acid content. This also is the reason that pears are rather constipating.

Plums. Plums and prunes are also very high in

calcium and sugar, especially when they are very ripe. They have a solvent effect on catarrhs of the digestive tract. All stony fruits such as prunes, apricots, peaches, etc., should be eaten with the peelings. They should be cleaned with a dry towel unless they have been sprayed. If so, they should be washed in cold water. The peels have a stimulating effect on the intestinal peristalsis.

Cherries are rich in iron and contribute to the formation of blood. Pie cherries are hard to digest on account of acid which is not burned up so easily as in citrus fruits. They stimulate the excretions of the organism.

Blackberries produce perspiration and dissolve mucus.

Strawberries dissolve uric acid deposits and are indicated for gout, rheumatism and migraine. They also contain phosphorus. Strawberries are better eaten raw because, contrary to other fruits, their fiber becomes toughened by cooking. It may be of interest to know that a certain disease, the Indian Sprue, can be cured only with a diet of fresh strawberries. Probably they contain a vitamin of a nature unknown to us as yet. There are certain people who show an idiosyncrasy or allergy against strawberries by reacting with a skin rash.

Grapes have a high sugar and acid content (vinous acid). Because of their sugar content (25%) they are used in most grape-growing countries as a food more than as a fruit. Four pounds of ripe sweet grapes contain 2,500 calories.

Huckleberries are useful in diarrhea, but only if

the juice is boiled. On the other hand, the old saying that huckleberry tea is good for diabetes has no foundation.

Raspberries, Gooseberries and Red Currants stimulate the activity of the kidneys. Black currants have a soothing effect on catarrh of the mucous membranes.

Oranges. Fresh orange juice is extremely important on account of its combination of sugar and acid, its high vitamin content and its alkaline effect on the urine.

Lemons. The lemon is very poor in sugar and very rich in organic acids. Its juice contains on an average of 7% citric acid. While it is very useful in the kitchen for flavoring purposes, it may be harmful to drink it concentrated. It has a caustic effect on the mucous membranes of the stomach and esophagus and is decalcifying to the enamel of the teeth and may even lead to poisoning. As a precipitant for calcium and for its relation to this mineral, it is discussed in the chapter on Salt and Calcium. The vitamin in lemon is so concentrated that minute amounts of this juice are sufficient to provide for our needs. The etheric oil which is contained in the lemon peel produces severe headaches if taken even in very small amounts.

Grapefruit stands in between oranges and lemons.

Pineapple juice is a mild and effective laxative. It contains a protein-splitting ferment, a quality for which it should be used by people who have a lack of hydrochloric acid and especially with a meal high in proteins.

Bananas are imported from tropical countries. Their meat is somewhat similar to that of the potato. The difference is that a ripe banana contains pure sugar instead of starch. On account of this high sugar content it is the most nutritious of all fruits. Two pounds of banana meat will satisfy the need for food for twenty-four hours.

Dates are known for their high sugar content and are therefore very nutritious. The French physiologist, Metschnikoff, recommended them on the theory that they prolonged life. They serve many people in the desert as a main food, especially in Northern Africa.

Figs should be recommended fresh as well as dried for their high alkaline content. They have a mild laxative effect. Good results have been reported lately concerning their use in the treatment of gallstone patients.

Corinths. Finally, a few words should be said about corinths, or dried seedless grapes, in contrast to dried seedy grapes, the raisins. Although growing in this country in large amounts and available at a very cheap price, they are not appreciated as to their full merits. All bio-chemists agree as to their high dietetic value.

Although the corinth loses certain aromatic qualities on the way from the fresh to the dry state, it gains others even more valuable.

In contrast to the grape, the corinth is poor in water (79.1% to 25.3%) while the sugar content is much higher (25% to 67.9)%.) All the alkaline minerals prevail in the corinth, which therefore is an excellent alkalinizing fruit. On account of the high sugar content it is very nourishing and because of its high cellulose content it is useful as a stimulant for the bowels.

The corinth should not only be used as an addition to salads and desserts, but as a regular food. It is especially important as a food between meals. There are very few people who dislike the taste of the corinth. For all those who indulge in sports, mountain climbing, hunting, etc., the corinth is best suited as a food to be taken between meals. It is more suitable for children than candy.

The medical value of the corinth, in a fresh as well as a dry state, was well known in ancient times. The name *passula* occurs quite frequently in the writings of the Roman historians. The corinth, as a food, has only advantages and is so cheap that it can be recommended for wide use to every one.

X

SPICES AND SPICY VEGETABLES

In every book on nutrition, one can find the caution that excessive use of pepper and spices causes an irritation of the stomach and mucous membranes of the intestines. This is true also of the mucous membranes of the upper respiratory tract. In questioning intelligent patients, one can often hear that they cannot fall asleep after a meal which has been highly seasoned. The nose chokes up and they have to change the side on which they lie in bed in order to clear the nasal passages for breathing. This is especially important in nervous cases. They wake up in the morning with a dry mouth and a bad breath. I know patients who, after eating highly seasoned dishes, must sneeze for a long time.

Condiments used sparingly do no harm. Indeed, they flavor the food and digestion is better when the food tastes good and is enjoyed. They have, of course, no food value.

The use of condiments and flavoring extracts to disguise spoiled or adulterated food is, of course, to be condemned.

We have briefly discussed the most common fruits, so let us now go on to the most common spices and spicy vegetables.

Celery has an abundance of alkaline minerals and should be used frequently by people who show a tendency toward acidosis. On account of its content of apiol, it has, if eaten in large amounts, an irritating effect on the kidneys. It should be avoided in kidney diseases. It may be well to mention here that the roots of celery have the same qualities as the stalks, but on account of their stronger content of apiol have more flavor. They make an excellent vegetable and a still better salad.

Onions. All kinds of onions are irritating to the mucous membranes. They stimulate the secretions of the stomach. In kidney diseases they should not be given. However, raw and cooked they are very useful in the kitchen as flavoring.

Radishes in all forms contain much alkaline minerals and a large amount of cellulose. The juice of radishes has been used for centuries against inflammations.

Asparagus has, in spite of its peculiar flavor, which goes into the urine, no bad effects on the kidneys and can be used by every one.

Rhubarb. The stalks do not contain the constituents of the leaves and roots. They have a laxative effect and if taken in large amounts may even lead to poisoning. But even the stalks should be used with caution in acid conditions on account of their content of oxalic acid (about 1.5%).

Cucumber. Any one who feels his stomach burdened when he eats raw cucumber should eat it steamed or in the form of a sauce. In intestinal catarrhs (diarrhea) it should be avoided.

Caraway seed is a valuable spice for bread and can be used without harm.

Cinnamon is one of the most useful spices, especially for desserts and has no harmful effects.

Ginger is less harmless and acts as an irritant on the kidneys.

Curcuma is a spice extracted from the root of an East Indian plant. It renders the characteristic flavor of the various brands of Worcestershire sauces. Due to its acid constituents it should be avoided in acid conditions, kidney diseases and irritations of the mucous membranes.

Pepper irritates all mucous membranes and the kidneys but used in small amounts just for flavoring it is harmless.

Paprica is still more irritating than pepper.

Mustard. The oil of mustard is one of the strongest irritants for the skin and mucous membranes we know. If brought in contact with the skin, it produces inflammation and vesiculation. If taken in larger amounts internally it inhibits the secretion of the digestive ferments and disturbs the digestion of proteins. It also irritates the kidneys. Mustard, pepper and paprica should be avoided, especially during the age of puberty because they all have an irritating effect on the sex organs. The dark French mustard contains less salt than the English yellow.

There are a number more of harmless spices which can and should be used in diets on account of their high flavoring qualities as chives, parsley, dills, cloves, bay leaf, mint, porree, marjoram, thyme, estargon, watercress, dandelion and many others.

Finally, let us mention **Yeast** not only for its high content of vitamin B, but also for its valuable protein. It should be used from time to time by every one. It is really not only a ferment but also a spice on account of its peculiar flavor.

XI

FATS

BUTTER is the principal fat used in this diet. It is not only necessary to provide energy (calories), but is very important for its vitamins.

It should be taken without salt. *Only sweet butter should ever be used.* The content of vitamins is richest during the spring and summer seasons because the cows eat germinating plants full of lecithin. The valuable parts of plants wilt later in the summer leaving only herbs for food, which contain much less lecithin. The hay is still less valuable in vitamins after the harvest, and very few vitamins remain in dry stable food. It can be seen how important it is that the animals, also, must have living food if we expect them to give milk and butter full of life. Generally speaking, all fats are comparatively poor in vitamins. Vitamin A is found in egg yolks and cod-liver oil; the anti-ricket vitamin D is found in fresh nut oils.

Not all parts of plants and animals are equally rich in vitamins. Among the plants, the germinating parts such as the seeds, contain most of the vitamins on account of their content of lecithin, cholesterol and other substances. These substances are found most concentrated wherever new life originates, for instance, a new branch, leaf, blossom or fruit. In these parts all are collected from the total plant, so that new life can develop. In this way the mystery of nature preserves the vitality and, under certain circumstances, puts new life in motion. Little, if any, of these substances are found in the roots, whose main task consists of sapping new substances from the soil.

Uncivilized people always prefer fresh, raw fat. In southern countries olive or nut oil is used more than any other.

The fats and oils have a stimulating effect on the production of bile and the pancreatic juice. The fats increase peristalsis and act as a lubricant for an easy bowel movement.

The digestibility of fats depends upon various factors; first, the melting point; second, whether the fat is fluid and saponifies well, and, finally, to what degree it resists the digestive ferments.

Food prepared with too much fat remains in the stomach for a long time and slows down the physiological time of digestion. The easiest fat to digest is fresh butter and fresh vegetable oil (olive oil). None of the other fats compare with these two as far as the important factors are concerned.

Canned or preserved fats should never be taken, with the exception of olive oil.

XII

SALT AND CALCIUM

CONTRARY to most salts, table salt contains no oxygen and consists only of the metal sodium and the acid-former chlorine (chemical formula NaCl). While the body makes use of the sodium by exchanging it for other alkalies, we have no use for the chlorine as a body builder. There is no organic matter in our system containing chloride. Wherever this acid-former is found in the organism, it is bound to a metal.

The importance of table salt lies in a different direction. Proteins, insoluble in pure water, for instance those of the blood, are kept in solution if the water contains a certain concentration of salt (0.05 to 0.1%). Furthermore salt is necessary to keep the osmotic tension of the body fluids at a normal level.

Minerals may be divided into two groups, those which taste alkaline and those which taste acid. These two types have opposite characteristics, and if brought together, form salts. These salts have a salty taste and do not change the color of litmus paper, which indicates their neutrality. To demonstrate this the following experience, which was reported in a medical journal may be given as an illustration: A girl intended to commit suicide by drinking lysol. She had heard of another case, where the drinking of lysol did not kill the person, but crippled her. In order to make sure that she would be killed, she added an equal amount of concentrated hydrochloric acid to the lysol. This mixture tasted terrible, but had the surprising effect that the girl did not even become very sick. After her stomach was washed out, she recovered within a few days. The explanation for this is that the amount of hydrochloric acid she used accidentally happened to balance the amount of lysol and therefore neutralized its action.

In diluted solution—in life and nature we deal only with diluted solutions—these salts are broken up into particles, which are loaded with electricity, the ions. The ions are the carriers of a tension, which they exert upon the cellular walls from within as well as from the outside. The tension from within must be the same as from the outside if a flow of fluid is to be avoided. This is the case at a concentration of approximately 0.9%. A solution of 0.9% sodium chloride in distilled water is called physiological salt or saline solution. As soon as the tension within the solution in which the cells are suspended increases, the cells expel fluid and shrink. On this principle rests the preserving power of table salt. Salted meat dries out and becomes an inadequate medium for the propagation of bacteria, which need moisture. The opposite happens if the tension within the cells becomes lower than that within the fluid in which they are suspended. This makes them swell and they become hydropic or water-logged.

Finally we find chlorine as a constituent of the hydrochloric acid (HCl), which is excreted by the mucous membrane of the stomach as an important agent of the digestive phase. This hydrochloric acid, however, does not become lost in the system, because it is absorbed again in the intestines after its transformation into sodium chloride. The gastric juice contains about 0.2 to 0.4% hydrochloric acid, which amounts under normal conditions to about 0.7 to 1.0 gm per day, depending on the food which has to be digested. The formation of hydrochloric acid naturally depends on the intake of sodium chloride. If too much salt is taken, the amounts of acid in the stomach will increase and produce hyper-acidity. This is very frequently the case with people who eat huge amounts of salt. These people need often to take sodium bicarbonate or any of its supplements after a meal, which will only temporarily neutralize the acid. If instead they would restrict the intake of salt they would have no need for alkalines after the meal.

We see that the actual need for table salt is very little. 1½ to 2½ gm per day, depending on the body weight, is the estimated need of the body, according to H. Strauss, an authority in this field. This alone shows that the organism receives quite enough salt, if its consumption is limited to what is contained in natural food. The fact that we consume very much more than is actually needed can be explained only by the habit of using it to such an extent that we find unsalted food unpalatable. Table salt is no food.

It is only an addition to food. The English language has no word for the German "Genussmittel," which expresses this best. Like nicotine, alcohol, coffee, tea and opiates, salt leads to a craving, and a large number of people do not want to eat even sweet fruits, coffee or chocolate without it. The restaurants know this craving for salt and serve most dishes salted accordingly. People who consume around 20 to 25 gm of salt per day, accumulate, in spite of the elimination through the urine, so much of it in their tissues, that they can be looked upon as living pickles. Expert biochemists have stated that an amount of salt exceeding 8 gm per day is injurious to the full utilization of proteins. Furthermore, we find salt in large amounts detrimental to the water economy in our system because of the fact that one gram of salt, in order to remain in solution, retains 70 gm of water in the body. A person can easily carry one to one and a half gallons of water retained by salt in the body without showing swellings.

We know of people who live without salt and never have known the use of it. They become sick on even small amounts of salt. Travelers and explorers have often reported this fact. People whose language knows no word for salt are the East Finns, the Kamtschadales, the Tunguses and Kirgises, the Tudas, some Arabian tribes, the Samoans, the Bushmen, the shepherds of South American Pampas and Fire Islands, the natives of New Holland and the Fiji Islanders. In this connection it may be interesting to know that the above-mentioned Kirgises live on the border of the salt steppes of Central Asia. Some of these people eat a great deal of sea-water fish, but the Tunguses, the Bedouins and the Fire Islanders do not even eat these. They are satisfied to get the necessary salt out of vegetable food alone.

Explorers have reported that certain people eat the ash of plants which contain much salt, and because of this, they called them salt-hungry people. The truth is that these people live in the desert and are hungry for plants on account of their need for alkaline minerals. These plants are not any richer in salt than others, but contain an abundance of mineralic alkali. All these people, like the Bushmen, the Hereros, the Akkas and others, are hunting tribes, who live principally on meat and therefore feel the need for alkalis.

The modern treatment which deprives patients with high blood pressure and kidney diseases of table salt is the best proof that man can get along without it. No one was ever harmed by taking too little or no salt, but an army of sick people live amongst us, who show the consequences of eating too much. In cases of suppuration and exudation too much salt counteracts recovery. Gerson and Sauerbruch have lately called attention to these facts and have proved that certain diseases such as migraine and tuberculosis of the skin can be improved and often cured by the reduction of salt alone.

The therapeutic effects of salt restriction are tremendous. First, this can be seen most effectively in dealing with inflammations, swellings and œdema, whether limited to an organ or generalized. Through its dehydrating effect it will also counteract the tendency toward suppuration and exudation. Secondly, the effects of calcium will become relatively evident; and thirdly, it will spare the work of the kidneys, favoring the elimination of certain metabolic products as for instance indican, uric acid and ketonbodies.

The effect of the restriction of salt on calcium is of utmost importance, and a few words must be said about it, as this problem is as yet little understood.

If sodium is eliminated in the intake, the biological effect of calcium in relation to inflammatory reactions will be enforced and the diet will work antiphlogistically. Sodium has a stronger affinity than calcium for the tissues, especially for the skin and mucous membrane. If large amounts of sodium chloride are taken, a great deal of it will be retained in the skin, mucous membrane, and other tissues and calcium will be expelled. Therefore, the sodium retained in the tissues will diminish the effect of calcium, which is needed in the body. On the other hand, with the reduction of sodium chloride, the calcium action will prevail and show its effect by counteracting inflammation. If a diet rich in calcium minerals is given, it is as a rule, not necessary to give additional calcium as a drug. But whenever this seems necessary, certain rules should be followed.

In order to understand the biochemical side of it, we have to go back a little further. The influence of alkaline or acid food on the assimilation of basic minerals was first brought out in 1912 by Luithlen, who found the following: If one feeds two rabbits, one with green leafy food and the other with oats, then examines the relation of the fed kations (sodium, potassium, calcium, magnesium) to those which have been eliminated in stools and urine, it will be found that the various kations replace themselves in the organism in equivalent amounts. This means: if an animal absorbs a given quantity of one kation, a corresponding amount of another kation must be eliminated. If we feed an animal two units each of sodium, potassium, magnesium and calcium and find the same quantities of each kation in the excretions, it must be concluded, that there was no absorption.

In a second experiment the same amount of kations were given, but the fed quantities of sodium and potassium did *not* appear in the excretions. This showed that they were absorbed. The analysis of the calcium and magnesium content of the stool and urine showed, in this experiment, a considerable increase above the intake. This proves, that the various kations may replace each other. If the figures found in the analysis are expressed in equivalent weights, we find that the replacement of the kations takes place in equivalent amounts.

Magnesium and calcium each have the chemical valency 2, hence, 1 molecule of calcium or magnesium will be expelled by 2 molecules of sodium or potassium, if the latter are assimilated. In other words, the reaction of single kations on one another, will always be equivalently balanced. The same principle has been observed in halogens. We know by biochemical experiments that the chlorine of the gastric juice can be displaced by bromine or iodine.

During the post-war period, Eppinger and I studied together the calcium metabolism and its relation to the other kations in normal cases, arthritic cases, and in cases of malnutrition due to the post-war nutritional conditions in Central Europe. People at that time suffered from a lack of minerals as the food supply was very short and fresh food, even meat, was very scarce. They developed diseases known as hunger œdema and osteoporosis, which disturbed the calcium metabolism significantly. Following are three characteristic results from a large series of experiments, which were done in the following way:

A normal person was fed for a period of ten days on a diet of a known calcium and magnesium content with the addition of 6 gm of sodium chloride per day. At the end of this period the stools and urine were examined for the calcium and magnesium content. For the next ten days the patient was fed on the same diet with an addition of 30 gm sodium chloride per day. At the end of this period the calcium and magnesium content of the stools and urine were again examined. For the following ten days he was fed on the same diet, returning to the additional 6 gm sodium chloride of the first period, and again the stools and urine were examined for sodium and calcium.

The diet which was given represented food on which the population in these countries had to live for approximately two years (1917 to 1919). This food consisted of condensed milk, flour, rice, eggs, margarine, cakes, sugar and marmalades. As a beverage, wine and mineral water were used. The following table shows the results of the examination in a normal person:

NORMAL PERSON

Amount of Sodium given daily for periods of 10 days each	Elimination of				Total Calcium	Total Magnesium	Results of increased intake of sodium
	Calcium		Magnesium				
	Urine	Stools	Urine	Stools			
1. 6 gm. sodium	0.1831	0.7782	0.1964	0.4705	0.9613	0.6674	Increased loss of calcium during sodium period 5.9% Magnesium 7.04%
2. 30 gm. sodium	0.2334	0.7854	0.1953	0.5668	1.0188	0.7621	
3. 6 gm. sodium	0.2345	0.8434	0.2329	0.4602	1.0779	0.6931	

In a second experiment a subacute arthritic patient was examined in the same way. He suffered from typical arthritic complaints and constipation, hyperacidity of the stomach, headache, chronic tonsillitis and repeated colds and sore throat.

The table on page 82 gives the results of the calcium and magnesium examination.

A third experiment concerned a patient of 64 years with typical complaints of osteoporosis, who had been living for the last two years exclusively on bread, potatoes and marmalade. The table on page 83 shows the results of the metabolic examination.

In another series of examinations sodium bicarbonate was given instead of sodium chloride. The results were similar to those in which sodium chloride was used, making it probable that not the molecule sodium chloride but rather the kation sodium is to blame for the action on the calcium. Later examinations, especially those of Falta, have shown in biochemical research that the action of sodium chloride rests primarily upon the kation sodium, and not, as previously thought, on the anion chlorine. While sodium chloride (NaCl) acts as a water absorbent, calcium chloride ($CaCl_2$) and potassium chloride (KCl) have a dehydrating effect, although both contain the anion Cl. From this point of view Falta and his co-workers have initiated experiments with a diet containing a salt mixture without sodium. The results of the application of this diet have not as yet been published.

Calcium became the center of interest as soon as

RHEUMATIC PERSON

| Amount of Sodium given daily for periods of 10 days each | Elimination of | | | | Total Calcium | Total Magnesium | Results of increased intake of sodium |
| | Calcium | | Magnesium | | | | |
	Urine	Stools	Urine	Stools			
1. 6 gm. sodium	0.2000	0.5328	0.0428	0.3961	0.5528	0.4389	Increased loss of calcium during sodium period 26.1%
2. 30 gm. sodium	0.0431	0.6630	0.0165	0.4049	0.6871	0.4914	
3. 6 gm. sodium	0.0270	0.3504	0.0223	0.3551	0.3774	0.3204	

PATIENT WITH OSTEOPOROSIS

| Amount of Sodium given daily for periods of 10 days each | Elimination of | | | | Total Calcium | Total Magnesium | Results of increased intake of sodium |
| | Calcium | | Magnesium | | | | |
	Urine	Stools	Urine	Stools			
1. 6 gm. sodium	0.1573	0.1377	0.0848	0.1925	0.2950	0.2773	Increased loss of calcium during sodium period 86.6% Magnesium 23.1%
2. 30 gm. sodium	0.1667	0.3827	0.0637	0.2777	0.5504	0.3414	
3. 6 gm. sodium	0.0991	0.1864	0.0412	0.0800	0.2855	0.1212	

it was realized how important a rôle it plays in the growth of bones. Its lack in rickets, for instance, is only a symptom and not the cause of rickets. The cause has first to be removed before calcium can act. Only together with cod-liver oil will calcium be effective, but then it is indispensable for recovery. It also was discovered that the insufficient calcium content of the tissues and blood favors the tendency toward inflammatory diseases. Here also it is not sufficient to have the patient take calcium-containing drugs, without paying attention to other factors. The daily need of calcium seems to lie between 1 and 2½ gm. How much of it is really assimilated, we do not yet know. This seems to depend on the amounts of other alkaline minerals simultaneously taken, as potassium, sodium, manganese as well as phosphorus and magnesium. So far we seem to know only that sodium slows down the assimilation of calcium, while potassium accelerates it.

Calcium is mostly given in the form of calcium chloride, calcium lactate or calcium gluconate. Calcium chloride is in some respects dangerous, especially in heart patients. Calcium gluconate is rather expensive. Whenever I found it necessary to give calcium with the diet to patients with frequent colds (especially children), I advised calcium carbonate. A dose of 2 to 2½ gm per day is sufficient, has no bad effects and will do just as well as the other far more expensive preparations. In some people it may be followed by constipation; if so, the following mixture is advisable: Four parts of calcium carbonate and one part calcium sulphate, about 2 gm per day. In this form it will stimulate the activity of the bowels and work as a mild laxative.

Some attention in relation to the calcium metabolism must be paid to the water of the district where the patient is living. Wherever one has to deal with soft water (calcium poor) some calcium should be given in addition to the diet.

As outlined before, the secret of the calcium action seems to lie in the relation of calcium within the food to other minerals, especially sodium, magnesia and phosphorus. Whenever any of these minerals are present in our food in too large amounts, the action of calcium will be impaired. (Examinations of Roese and R. Berg.)

A word may be said here about the abundant use of citrus fruits in relation to calcium. Like everywhere else, so here, too much may be as harmful as not enough. Years ago, Von Noorden showed that citric acid precipitates calcium and makes it ineffective. The enforcement of the calcium action against inflammation by natural ways is one of the main principles of our diet. If large amounts of citric acid are taken, the effect of this principle will be lessened. It is in my opinion unnecessary to drink huge amounts of orange juice and grapefruit juice in order to provide the organism with vitamin C. For this purpose minute amounts are sufficient. In cases where calcium as a drug is given, citrus fruits should be left out for about four to five hours after the calcium is given. The second reason for which citrus juices are given is their alkaline effect on metabolism. This alkaline effect can be produced just as well with other fruit or vegetable juices. I, therefore, advise the reduction in the amount of orange and grapefruit juices to some extent. This should be remembered especially in cases suspected of calcium deficiency. The problem is different when quick action against acidosis is needed, as in very acute conditions or before and after an anæsthetic.

Sinus patients only rarely present a condition where such quick action is needed. On the contrary, the effect of the diet will be increased with a gradual but persistent transmineralization.

The American dietary is probably more deficient in calcium than in other minerals. This deficiency of calcium can never be counteracted by taking certain calcium salts in the form of patent medicine, as advertised. Here, as everywhere in nature, the life-giving principle rests upon the natural state in which calcium is taken.

Some people may object to the restriction of sodium chloride, pointing to the fact that animals, for instance, often make vigorous efforts to visit the salt licks, which cattle, deer and even horses seem to find necessary to their health and comfort. In view of this, let me impress the fact that no one has ever said that sodium in the form of sodium chloride is not necessary to health. The trouble is, that most people consume about twenty gram or more daily, which is approximately ten times as much as is needed for the body requirements.

In the kitchen "just a pinch" of salt is used with everything, and at the table salt is often added in amounts which remind one of the salt licks of animals. One receives the impression that people who do that, do not care what they eat, because they cover the taste of every dish to the extent that a distinction between good or bad food becomes impossible. With the advised diet, the intake of sodium chloride will be between 4 to 5 gm a day, still leaving a comparatively large reserve for the organism, and this amount can easily be obtained from natural sources.

The diet that I advise for sinus patients should not be called a salt-free diet, because it is not free of salt. The appropriate name would be salt-poor. Practically all the salt taken is contained in the natural food. The following table published by Wolff-Eisner in the *Medical World* shows an analysis of a salt-poor diet as it is given in the Clinic of Sauerbruch. The amounts of the various foods correspond approximately to what I have given my patients:

SODIUM CHLORIDE INTAKE PER WEEK

600 gr.	Meat	= 6x100 mg =	600 mg	Sodium	Chloride
10,000	Milk	= 10x1600	=16,000	"	"
700	Eggs	= 7x84	= 588	"	"
300	Rice	= 3x55	= 165	"	"
200	Wheat	= 2x96	= 192	"	"
100	Peas	=	= 100	"	"
500	Whipping cream	= 5x130	= 650	"	"
1,000	Bread	= 10x500	= 5,000	"	"
1,600	Potatoes	= 16x76	= 1,230	"	"
3,500	Fruits	=100x35	= 3,500	"	"
3,500	Vegetables	=100x35	= 3,500	"	"
Sum			31,585 mg		

This figure divided by seven indicates an average daily consumption of 4.5 gm sodium chloride. If in addition to that, the consumption of two glasses of vegetable juice, which is often advised, is added, with an approximate salt content of about 0.5 gm per day, we arrive at a total of 5 gm per day.

XIII

WATER ECONOMY

It is hardly necessary to drink water with the following diet. In cooking vegetables, butter or oil should be used instead of water. Fruit salads, vegetables, milk, fruits and vegetable juices and occasionally a cup of coffee or tea, provide sufficient water. The little water, which must be used to soak the dried fruits and vegetables during the winter, should only replace the water lost during the drying process. On hot days during the summer, and with hard labor in the winter, an additional amount of water may be needed. As a rule the patients report that they perspire much less after taking the diet than they did before, a fact easily explained by the restriction of table salt. Large circles still believe that it is healthful to consume a great quantity of water. Aschner and others have shown again and again, that large amounts of water do not agree with the stomach after a period of time. In the majority of cases, it is followed by a dilation of the stomach, which is often felt as a pressure and uncomfortable tension in the abdomen.

It may be quite difficult to convince a housewife that soups are entirely unnecessary in our diet. This is especially true of meat broth, which is nothing but a watery solution of non-nutrient substances.

The food eaten by animals is split up in the digestive tract into different parts. Most of these are assimilated while others are not. Some of these substances are normally carried by the circulating blood from the places where they have been deposited in muscles, bones and connective tissues, to the kidneys where they are excreted in a watery solution, the urine. Almost the same substances are extracted from animal meats and bones in meat broth.

The only difference between meat broth and excretions lies in the comparatively little change to which these substances are subjected on the way to and through the kidneys. The idea that these substances are valuable is a very old one. We know that in the Middle Ages, as even today in Oriental countries, animal urine was used as a medicine and drink against certain diseases. All these substances have a stimulating effect on the nervous system. Because we know that stimulation does not mean an increase in strength but rather an increased deterioration of the nervous system, we should give up the illusion that meat soups are essential to our health.

Large amounts of fluid naturally may be necessary after prolonged perspirations or diarrhea. Fluids then should be taken in the form of mild teas or fruit juices, rather than in the form of ice-cold water.

For centuries man knew that the earth contained part of the necessary remedies against disease. These remedies they sought to find in mineral waters. Out of this concept the habit of drink-cures developed.

It should be said here, that natural mineral water will lose part of its effect, if bottled. If any effect can be expected from such a cure, it must be taken at its natural source. The natural waters, even when bottled, are still superior and more effective than the artificial waters, which never can replace nature.

XIV

THE DIETETIC THERAPY

A DIETETIC treatment should always be worked out by a physician who is familiar with the patient. In treating irritations, catarrhs and suppurations of the nasal mucous membranes, similar rules will have to be followed to those used in the successful dietetic therapy of diseases which very frequently accompany sinus diseases. For rheumatism, arthritis, neuritis, constipation, headaches and certain skin diseases a number of authorities have emphasized the great importance of diet. Widal, Pemberton, Sansum, Jarvis, von Noorden, Gerson, Sauerbruch, Urbach, and a great many others have advised diets for these ailments. In pointing out this fact, I want to emphasize that, using similar principles, the diet which I have successfully advised for so many patients with sinus diseases, is no new discovery. It simply applies old experiences in a new field.

The principles of the diet consist firstly, in the restriction of salt, and secondly, in choosing the food in such a way as to counteract acidosis. The diet must be an alkaline one. Its main characteristics are the following:

1. The use of only fresh food.
2. The restriction of salt.

3. The preference of alkaline food.
4. The reduction of animal proteins.
5. The reduction of carbohydrates.
6. The use of unrefined carbohydrates whenever possible.

The most difficult part of this diet lies in the restriction of salt. For most people it seems to be difficult to break the habit of salting food, especially when they are ignorant of the method of preparing food tastily without salt. In the appendix, a variety of cooking recipes will be found which may be a help in overcoming this difficulty. These recipes are not theoretical, but are the result of eight years of actual experience in cooking and eating according to the principles of the diet. Several substitutes for salt have been suggested, at least until the patient has become accustomed to the food. I find that Curtasal fulfills this purpose best. It does not need to be measured and can be used in the kitchen as well as on the table. The often-mentioned vegetable salt cannot be used, as it is table salt with an addition of vegetable minerals. Curtasal should be used moderately and the patient should be informed that it is given only temporarily until he has become adjusted to the diet.

Alkaline drugs should be avoided. I never needed to resort to sodium bicarbonate, magnesium usta, or bisodol and others, even for patients whose acid condition was very noticeable. The diet is such that the production of too much acid in the stomach will be counteracted in a natural way. In cases where there is a lack of hydrochloric acid in the stomach, care should be taken not to reduce salt too strictly. However, I have never come across such a case in relation to sinus diseases, and we do not need to be concerned with this group.

To children and in certain cases where it seems necessary, cod-liver oil should be given. I usually prescribe phosphorated cod-liver oil, decreasing the phosphorous content after three or four weeks.*

For the use of calcium drugs, see the chapter on Salt and Calcium.

The diet is directed to counteract acidosis, to increase the effect of calcium in the system and to prevent an eventual lack of vitamins.

Some of the effects of the diet are hard to explain as long as we have no more exact knowledge of the so-called acidotic conditions. It is difficult sometimes to prove scientifically that certain food combinations are deleterious and others helpful. Clinical observations, however, have always been and always will be recognized as an important means of attaining medical knowledge. This is particularly true of dietetic knowledge. When a physician repeatedly gets excellent results while following a particular line of treatment, he is justified in concluding that his method is sound, in spite of the fact that he may not be able thoroughly to prove his thesis by biochemical or physiological laboratory methods.

---

* Rx   Phosphorus 0.02
       Ol. jecoris aselli
                     300,00
       Sig:
           one teaspoon full 2-3 x p. d.

XV

APPLICATION OF THE DIET

In applying this diet some people may find that they have to concentrate their thoughts considerably on how, when and what to eat. All those who suffer from frequent colds, influenza, sinus suppurations and their consequences, rheumatism, neuritis and headaches, sooner or later come to the conclusion that it will be much better in the end to submit to certain rules concerning their living and eating habits, than to be a steady paying guest at the doctor's office.

It is natural that only a schedule can be given in a book. It will fulfill its purpose if it gives such advice as can be carried out by the majority of people. Expensive and time-consuming measures will be restricted to the utmost. The diet as outlined in this book will have to be varied by the physician as to the individual needs and circumstances of the patient. Very sick, bed-ridden patients, patients with fever, convalescent patients and children, will each have to be treated differently. All those, who constitutionally are subject to colds and sinus diseases, are in a group by themselves, and have to keep to this diet in order to prevent rather than to cure. It will be a special problem to avoid setbacks which are bound to occur in people who have to eat in restaurants and those who have a great many social engagements which take them away from home cooking. Still more difficult is the problem with bachelors. In such cases a solution can be found only individually, otherwise they become victims of their professions or their habits. This is similar to the case of people who have found employment in tropical countries and cannot stand the climate. Never mind how good the position, the climate will not improve, nor will their health; they must give up one or the other.

On the other hand, my experiences have shown, that with some goodwill and intelligence, the principles of the diet can be applied to every one, whether he or she be a man of leisure, a hard-working business man or a sales girl in a department store. Every person, regardless of who he is or where he lives, must have time enough to prepare at least two good meals a day. If one lives under the illusion that he is so busy making a livelihood that he cannot afford to give this much time and thought to his health, he may just as well give up.

I have noticed during many years of experience, that all these patients, who have suffered for years, and spent a great deal of their money on hospitals, operations and doctor bills, or at health resorts, without the desired results, are only too glad to devote more time and thought to their food and its preparation.

The people of today do not give enough thought to their food as long as it is clean and satisfying.

No one should believe that civilization will ever reach the point where we can live on food in the form of pills. No machine, technique, discovery or invention can take us that far away from nature. About one hundred years ago Jean Jacques Rousseau expressed his famous *back-to-nature* philosophy. He applied it to thought and art only. Let us apply it to food.

XVI

WHAT TO EAT

THE advice concerning what to eat may first begin with what not to eat.

FORBIDDEN FOODS

Canned foods, table salt, salted butter, alcohol, candies, smoked meats and fish, bacon, ham, sausages, sardines, herring, caviar, etc. Also pickles, catsup, highly seasoned sauces (including bottled sauces), spiced cheeses, preserved olives, salted almonds, crackers, salt sticks and hot biscuits should be avoided.

FOODS PERMITTED IN LIMITED AMOUNTS

Meat, not over 500 gm or 16 ounces per week; in addition about 200 gm or 6 ounces per week of sweet bread, brain, kidneys, spleen, liver or fresh fish.

Seafood. Whatever seafood is taken it should be figured within the above-mentioned 200 gm per week. Crab, crawfish or lobster can be taken if bought alive and boiled in unsalted water.

Eggs. Two eggs per day, those used in mayonnaise, puddings, custards, creams and egg sauces included.

Grain Products. About 1 to 1½ ounces of grain

products a day. The flour used in cooking should be whole wheat and the bread should be rye, whole wheat, pumpernickel, or raisin bread containing lima bean or soy bean flour. One or two slices of zwieback may be used if necessary. If the advice is given to restrict salt entirely, salt free bread should be used. This can easily be made at home and the recipe will be found in the appendix.

Unpolished rice, tapioca, cream of wheat, oatmeal, lima and soy beans may be used if kept within the carbohydrate limit.

Potatoes. One potato should be eaten with every main meal, luncheon and dinner. It can be eaten in any form except fried, unless prepared according to the recipes on page 141 and following. Baked, mashed, scalloped, boiled, etc. will do.

Sugar. About one ounce of sugar may be used a day, preferably brown unrefined or raw sugar. Honey or maple syrup may be taken in addition.

Coffee—Tea. One cup of weak coffee is allowed for breakfast. Tea should also be weak and limited to one cup per day. Preferably a tea consisting of various herbs should be used. The tea that I prescribe for my patients consists of the following:

> Fol. malvae
> Fol. mellissae
> Fol. graminis
> Fol. camomile
> Fol. sarsaparillae
> Fol. salviae
> Hb. minth. pip. aa 30.00
> **Sign: Tea**

This tea provides plenty of alkaline minerals, favors diuresis, and because of its pleasant taste, is liked by the majority of patients. It provides a good substitute in winter where there is a shortage of fresh green vegetables. One or two cups of this tea should be taken every day.

FAVORED FOODS

Milk. One quart of milk should be consumed a day with the addition of one-half pint of cream. Raw milk should be taken if obtained from reliable cows. Buttermilk, kefir, yogurth, cottage cheese, Philadelphia cream cheese should be used freely.

Fats. From 3 to 4 ounces a day of fresh unsalted butter is sufficient. For salads and vegetables pure olive oil should be used freely.

Vegetables and Salads. All kinds of vegetables are left to the choice of the patient. These he can obtain in an ample variety at the vegetable markets throughout the year. He should not rely on what the grocer happens to have in stock for him.

Spices and Herbs. Full use may be made of all available herbs. Dill, porree, parsley, sage, rose-marin, cloves, mint, dandelion, endives, watercress, chives are good flavoring and refreshing herbs. In addition to these, marjoram, estragon, vanilla, cinnamon, nutmeg, bayleaf, allspice, onions in moderation, mushrooms, garlic, anis, caraway seed, French mustard, all kinds of nuts, raisins, and especially corinths, will contribute to the flavoring of food.

Fruits. Plenty of fresh and dried fruits should be taken. There is no objection to home-made pre-

serves, if they are made without the addition of
acids, and canned in glass jars. These preserves,
however, should not be older than one season. In
this form jam, marmalade and jelly can be used.
During the winter, when there is a shortage of fresh
fruit, dried fruit should be used. Dried apricots,
peaches, prunes, pears, raisins, figs, dates, etc., are
always available. Care should be taken that they
are unsulphured. If the absolute need for salt is felt,
Curtasal may be added to the food. For sick people,
who are either confined to bed before or after an
operation, or convalescent, and especially for children, the meals should be divided in the following
way:

7:30 A.M. *Breakfast:* Orange or any fruit juice. Oatmeal or cream of wheat, or tapioca with cream. One
slice of zwieback or rye bread with butter. One cup
of weak coffee.

9:30 A.M.: One glass of milk or vegetable or fruit juice.
One-half slice of bread and butter.

12:00 M. *Luncheon:* According to the menus with the
addition of one glass of milk and one-half glass of
fruit or vegetable juice.

4:00 P.M.: One glass of milk or vegetable or fruit juice.
One-half slice of bread and butter.

6-6:30 P.M. *Dinner:* According to the menus with the
addition of one glass of milk and one-half glass of
fruit or vegetable juice.
One-half hour before bed time, one cup of herb tea
should be taken as indicated above.

This division of the day has to be changed somewhat if the patient is working away from home. It

then has to be adapted to the individual needs as indicated in the previous chapter. A glass of milk or fruit juice between meals is good, if possible. A few raisins, nuts or an apple can easily be carried in the pocket and will make it possible for the busiest business man to follow the instructions to eat oftener than three times a day. A total amount of two to three glasses of fruit or vegetable juice must be consumed per day.

The drugs, which are at times prescribed with the diet, have been previously mentioned as to their nature and dosage.

XVII

WHEN TO EAT

It is hardly possible to give definite rules which can be applied to every one, as to the time of eating and how often to eat. Different races, different nations and people of different countries all eat at different times. It has been shown that under normal circumstances a person can get along very nicely and remain healthy with three meals a day. This applies to a moderate climate and to people of healthy constitution, but even here the opinions vary as to when the main meal should be eaten.

Should one eat a heavy breakfast or should one fast in the morning? Should the main meal be at noon or at vesper time? Theoretically, one seems to be justified in advising a heavy breakfast after the fasting during the night. Every activity of the body is greatly reduced during sleep; the glands practically cease secreting, the temperature reduces, and the metabolism is lowered. From this, however, it can be concluded, that due to the lower metabolism during the night there would still be enough reserves present in the morning to prevent the necessity of taking food. For the many people who do not seem to be able to eat as soon as they awaken, it will be better not to eat heavily in the morning.

If the evening meal is not taken too late, it is well to choose this time for the main meal, if for no other reason, than that business cannot deter one from taking time, not only to eat but also to enjoy the food.

In our case, however, we are not dealing with normal people or normal circumstances. As outlined before, all sinus patients show a tendency toward acidosis. Long intermissions between meals cause an accumulation of acid in the stomach, which gives the feeling of hunger. If the acid in the stomach reaches a certain point, it produces belching and heart-burn, which most people try to counteract by taking alkalies in the form of sodium carbonate, bisodol and many of the advertised drugs. If instead of this they would take a small amount of food between meals, as has been outlined in the detailed description of the diet, there would be no need to take these alkalies.

During starvation and in proportion to its severity, the body is sustained by the consumption of its own fat and protein. This gives rise to acidosis in varying forms of severity. An acidosis of this type in women was called by Sansum very descriptively, "shoppers' headache." Women become absorbed in shopping to the neglect of food. Acidosis develops with headache, bad breath and sometimes nausea.

Every American traveler, who has been in Europe, tells of his surprise in having seen the people in most countries eat five times or even oftener during the day. The reasons are many, but one of the consequences is that these people do not have so many colds and sinus diseases as people in this country. Eating oftener counteracts acidosis. In diseases, which are characterized by a profuse secretion of acid in the stomach, the method of feeding every two or three hours is accepted without objection by the medical profession as well as the laity, and people with ulcers and other disorders of the stomach are willing to submit to this rule. Why then should those suffering from sinus diseases say that they cannot submit to a diet, which forces them to eat oftener than three times a day? The only reason for this that I can see, is lack of information and education. While I advise patients to have their breakfast, luncheon and dinner at the usual time, I insist that they take something between meals, if it is nothing but a glass of milk or a slice of pumpernickel with cheese, which every one can find time to eat, even during office hours. If people would only realize how much unnecessary suffering is due to prejudice! How often does one hear the desire to be different, and how often does one see these same people afraid to be different?

If the main meal is eaten at six or six-thirty in the evening, something should be taken half an hour before bed time, if it is nothing but a glass of milk. Many patients complain of bad breath, and quite often this is due to an accumulation of acid in the stomach. Nearly every one has a bad breath when awakening, that being one of the reasons why we wash the mouth so thoroughly in the morning. After fasting for six or more hours the stomach is in the same condition as it is after a night's sleep of seven to eight hours.

The food eaten between meals does not need to be cooked and can consist of food which is always available. I insist that my patients eat between the three main meals. The complaint that children have no appetite, leave food on their plates and do not finish their meals, is a very common one. If children were fed small amounts of food frequently during the day, instead of forcing three big meals, much better results could be obtained.

XVIII

THE PREPARATION OF FOOD

THE patient must first be instructed that it is very important to use only fresh and unspoiled food and also that he has to expect an increase in his food budget from 10 to 12%, depending on the season.

In this chapter only the principles will be pointed out, as the details about the various dishes will be found under recipes.

Concerning the cooking of vegetables, special care must be used in order to avoid boiling, steaming, or in any way heating them too long. Not only the type of preparation, but also the time plays an important rôle. Nothing should be left on the stove or in the oven longer than is absolutely necessary. The gravest mistake which is made in the kitchen occurs during the cooking process. If the vegetables are boiled, the water must be used with the vegetables. If the water is thrown away, the minerals are lost and one eats vegetables which, depending on the length of time that they have been in the water, have turned more or less acid. Therefore, the preparation of vegetables is best done in the following way: Three to four tablespoons of water are added to the vegetables when they are put on the stove, just enough to keep them from burning; they should always be cooked in a covered container. After steaming for 20 to 25 minutes, olive oil or fresh butter should be added and the container left closed until the food is ready to be served. *No salt should be added.* The time of cooking depends on the vegetable, but from ¼ to ¾ of an hour should be enough for all varieties. The boiling point of fat is considerably lower than that of water, consequently not as much heat is needed as with water, and the vegetables will be cooked more quickly. If the steaming is done in this way, the aromatic as well as the mineralic substances will be retained and not extracted as with water. Also, the lack of salt will not be so noticeable. In preparing cabbage, cauliflower, onions and other aromatic vegetables, the odor can be eliminated by adding a small piece of bread while steaming.

Another method of avoiding the odor in certain vegetables consists of wiping off the first condensed water from the cover, which contains most of the aromatic substances. This should be done about five minutes after the steaming has begun.

Herbs, condiments, lemons, raw onions or garlic should not be steamed with the vegetables, but should be added at the end of the cooking period to spice and increase the flavor.

Freshly prepared vegetables, if they have been steamed only to the point of being done, may be warmed over once for dinner. It is detrimental to keep dishes warm on the stove over a long period of time. If for any reason this must be done, it will be better to remove them from the stove as soon as they are done and heat again when needed. Leftovers can be used in salads.

Leafy vegetables should be selected carefully, the wilted parts and blossoms separated and thrown away, while the remainder should be washed thoroughly and drained until nearly dry.

Root vegetables must not be peeled, but thoroughly cleaned in lukewarm water with a stiff brush and all spoiled spots removed. For sick people it may be advisable to grate or cut the vegetables into small particles. If prepared this way they will take less time to steam.

If legumes are used in the form of non-green dried beans, peas or lentils, care should be taken not to give too much in one meal as they produce bloating and considerable gas. One can avoid that, however, if about ½ teaspoon of sodium bicarbonate (sufficient for five servings) is added to the food while cooking.

All vegetables can be used in the form of purée if the condition of the patient demands.

FRUIT JUICES

The fruit juices should be a combination of several fruits. A combination of oranges, grapes, apples and various berries is most suitable. If desired a few drops of lemon juice may be added. Only fresh and fully ripe fruit should be used. Dried or canned fruits should not be used for juices. The fruit juices are more pleasant to drink, if first put through a sieve or cheesecloth to eliminate the seeds, pulp and

stones. Pears, plums and prunes are not so good as
the other fruits for juice. Canned *raw* fruit juices
are harmful because they may cause fermentation.

VEGETABLE JUICES

Similarly to Gerson I stress the importance of
fresh vegetable juices, because vegetables taken in
their natural state are satiating, and many patients
report being fed up with them and refuse to take
enough. In taking the juices they not only get the
most essential part of the vegetable, but at the same
time satisfy their thirst. In preparing these juices
cleanliness is absolutely necessary not only of the
vegetables, but also of the hands and containers;
otherwise fermentation may produce diarrhea. Only
the best and freshest vegetables should be used.
People who want to accumulate root vegetables as
root celery, beets or carrots can keep these over the
winter in moist sand. After two or three months
they become wilted, but by soaking in water for a
few hours can be freshened.

For the preparation of vegetable juice all vegetables must be carefully examined for spoiled spots
and wilted leaves. After being cleaned and drained,
they should be grated, then pressed through a fruit
press or ground through a meat grinder or pressed
through a clean towel or cheesecloth. For smaller
portions, sufficient for one or two persons, this can
easily be done by pressing the grated vegetables
through a gauze pouch (cheesecloth) Fig. 1. A fruit
press as shown in Fig. 2 is most satisfactory in pressing the juice out of all kinds of vegetables.

To obtain the juice from tubers, these should not be peeled, but brushed thoroughly until clean. Thereafter the same procedure as before mentioned should be followed. In hospitals and sanatoria

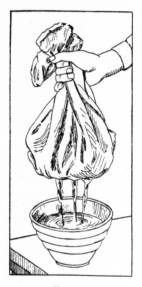

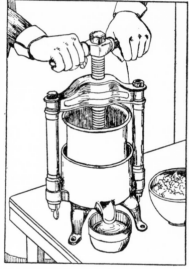

FIG. 1.

One obtains the fruit juice by pressing the juicy fruits through a cheesecloth.

FIG. 2.

In order to obtain the vegetable juice the grated vegetables are put through a fruit press of a type as shown in the picture.

the use of a large, electrical fruit press is advisable. In order to obtain various flavors an addition of small amounts of lettuce, watercress, radish and onion juice, which is prepared in the same way, can be used. It is best to mix all these vegetables in the desired proportions after the grating and press the juice out together.

MIXING THE JUICES

The amount of juices the patient should take should be decided on by the physician, depending on the fluid needs of the particular case. The juices are an essential part of the diet due to their high mineral and vitamin content. One may start with small amounts in order first to try the patient's digestive tract, but one should try to reach a daily average of at least one quart per day. Carrots, tomatoes, beets, spinach, lettuce, cabbage, celery and cauliflower are the most useful vegetables for this purpose. Orange, lemon and apple juice added, makes them very palatable. For very sick people warm oatmeal may be prepared with a small amount of juice. Tomato juice is the only vegetable juice which is palatable without an addition of other fruit juices. But it must be made from fresh tomatoes.

The prepared juices can be put in the refrigerator and kept for about eight hours, but after eight hours fermentation begins. Some of the fruit juices may ferment earlier as for instance, apple juice, which ferments after three hours. Fruit and vegetable juices must be kept separately and mixed only shortly before drinking. They should be cold when drunk. They should not be kept in aluminum or metal containers, because only glass or porcelain dishes will not alter their taste.

XIX

TESTING THE URINE FOR ACIDITY AND CHLORIDES

For those who are interested in this subject the book entitled, *The Determination of Ions*, by William Mansfield Clark, published by Williams & Wilkins Company, Baltimore, is recommended.

The normal hydrogen-ion concentration of the blood is 7.35 expressed as pH. Following a simple teaching interpretation of the logarithmic methods of expressing the hydrogen-ion concentration: The hydrogen-ion concentration of the normal blood is equal to the decimal fraction 0.00000004467. This is less than the hydrogen-ion concentration of distilled water, which is equal to the decimal fraction 0.0000001. Distilled water is neutral in its reaction. The blood having a lower hydrogen-ion concentration than distilled water is therefore slightly alkaline. The writing of such decimal fractions consumes time and space and is therefore inconvenient, hence the logarithmic method representing such fractions is used instead. All decimal logarithm are minus, hence the minus sign is dropped. The normal hydrogen-ion concentration of the blood is written as pH 7.35, which interpreted, means that the potential of the hydrogen-ion concentration of the blood is equivalent to a decimal fraction corresponding to the logarithm minus 7.3500.

A still simpler method of making the hydrogen-ion concentration expressions of urine acidity understandable to patients is, to express such acidity not in logarithms but in the number of times that the urine is more acid than normal blood, as in the following table:

Urine pH	Acidity Times That of Normal Blood	Urine pH	Acidity Times That of Normal Blood
7.35	1.0	5.80	35.4
7.30	1.1	5.70	44.6
7.20	1.4	5.60	56.2
7.10	1.7	5.50	70.8
7.00	2.2	5.40	89.1
6.90	2.8	5.30	112.2
6.80	3.5	5.20	141.3
6.70	4.4	5.10	177.8
6.60	5.6	5.00	223.8
6.50	7.0	4.90	281.8
6.40	8.9	4.80	354.8
6.30	11.2	4.70	446.7
6.20	14.1	4.60	562.3
6.10	17.7	4.50	708.0
6.00	22.3	4.40	891.2
5.90	28.1	4.35	1000.0

The reactions of the urine may easily be determined by means of dyes which are called indicators. For a long time pieces of paper dipped in litmus dye have been used for this purpose. This dye has the property of turning red in an acid solution and blue in an alkaline one. The dye litmus, however, is not a very delicate indicator and it is generally accepted that a urine which is acid enough to turn blue litmus paper red, is far too acid and a urine which is alkaline enough to turn red paper blue is probably too alkaline. More delicate dyes as Brom Thymol Blue and Methyl Red have, therefore, been chosen.

The dyes chosen have the advantage of changing to several colors depending upon the degree of alkalinity or acidity. The dye, Brom Thymol Blue (BTB) is yellow in a slightly acid solution and blue in a slightly alkaline solution. As the reaction changes from acid to alkaline, the color changes gradually from a yellow-green to a green, to a blue-green and finally to blue. The dye Methyl Red (MR) is used in the more acid urines. In extremely acid urine it is red and in moderately acid urine it is yellow, with varying color shades between.

There has been devised a new dye, called Duplex Indicator, which covers the range of the dyes BTB and MR, so that with their new simplified outfit only one dye need be used.* For the purpose of the practitioner the colorimetric method is sufficient.

The urine sample must be taken from a 24-hour urine sample. The patient is advised to collect his urine for 24 hours and use some thymol crystals in the container for the conservation of the urine. The container in which the urine is conserved, should not be bottled with a cork because this will turn the urine acid. If a cork stopper is used it must be soaked in melted paraffin. A clean rubber stopper is the best. The patient is advised to bring one ounce sample of the total amount of urine to the office the following day and the urine should be examined at

* From W. D. Sansum, *The Normal Diet,* 3rd Ed. Courtesy C. V. Mosby Co. (St. Louis), pp. 121-123.

once because by standing it will turn alkaline. The directions for the use of the hydrogen-ion concentration colorimeter are attached to every instrument and can be looked up in every textbook of laboratory methods that has been written within the last three or four years.

The examinations for chlorides are as important as for acidity, but do not need to be repeated so frequently. The estimation of the chlorides in the urine is best done by the *Larrson* method. Those who prefer, may use the method of Volhard, but as this latter method needs more reagents, some of which have to be freshly prepared, it is more expensive.

The principle of Larrson's method is as follows: The pigments, urates and other interfering substances are removed from the urine by absorption with blood charcoal. The chlorides are estimated in a measured amount of the filtrate by the direct titration with silver nitrate, using potassium chromate as an indicator. The reagents are:

1. Standard silver nitrate solution prepared by dissolving 29.063 gm of pure fused silver nitrate in distilled water and filling accurately to 1,000 gm. The solution should be kept in the dark.

1 c.c. corresponds to 0.01 gm NaCl (0.00606 gm Cl).

2. Merck's pure blood charcoal (Carbo Sanguinis puriss.). Ordinary animal charcoal is useless.

3. A 5% solution of potassium chromate.

Method of analysis. To 1 gm of the blood charcoal in a dry flask add 20 c.c. of the urine. Shake vigorously and repeat the shaking at intervals for 10

minutes. Filter through a small dry paper into a dry
tube. Measure 10 c.c. of the filtrate by means of a
pipette and transfer it to a small beaker. Add 5 or 6
drops of the chromate and titrate with the silver nitrate from a burette until the end point is reached,
as indicated by the appearance of a reddish-brown
color.

Calculation. 1 c.c. of silver=0.01 gm NaCl.
Example. 10 c.c. of the filtered urine required 10.6 c.c.
                of silver.
              So. 10 c.c contain 10.6x0.01 gm NaCl.
              So 100 c.c contain 1.06 gm NaCl.

Naturally also for this test the total amount of 24
hours urine has to be calculated. The patient should
be advised to collect the 24-hour urine sample,
measure it at home and bring 1 ounce to the office.
This way both the acidity as well as the chlorides
can be determined.

The normal chloride content of 24 hours lies
around 10 gm according to the latest research. This
is the figure for a normal person, who does not take
salt in excess. People can frequently be found, with
a content of 20 to 25 gm per day. This has often
been the case in my experience. The chloride content, after the application of the diet, should be reduced to 4 to 5 gm per day and kept there.

In testing the acidity of the urine, an alkaline
urine may be found sometimes when a very acid
urine should be expected according to clinical symptoms (hyperemia and congested mucous membranes,
ample suppuration) and history. In questioning

these patients, I found that within the last day or two they had taken large doses of sodium bicarbonate, or in other cases large amounts of citric fruit juices. Both naturally will turn the urine reactions quite alkaline, misleading the physician to believe that the patient is not suffering from acidity. Again questioning these patients, one will, as a rule, find that they have either lived on an acid diet or turned the vegetable food acid by preparing it the wrong way. According to my experience the best results will be obtained if the patient is managed so that his pH is kept around 7.1 to 6.5 The urine will then be two to seven times more acid than normal blood.

XX

HOW LONG SHALL THE DIET BE CONTINUED?

THIS question, which is often put to the physician, can be answered only in a broad way because the individual, constitutional and professional circumstances of the patient have to be considered.

If a high sodium chloride content is found in the urine, the diet is started more drastically in order to eliminate salt as fast as possible. This can be done by keeping the patient for one or two days entirely on a fruit and vegetable diet without milk, cheese, meat and carbohydrates. On the second and third day the regular diet is started. The patient is kept strictly on this diet for two or three months depending on his condition. Thereafter if his condition is improved or if he is well, small amounts of salt in the kitchen may be allowed once or twice a week. The use of salt on the table or the eating of excessively salty food should always be prohibited to these patients. A great number of them report that they do not miss the salt at all. Some even display a dislike for highly salted food, like sausages and ham, after they have refrained from salt for longer than two months. Patients whom I have kept free of colds for one and one-half to two years were allowed to go back to a normal diet, and were advised always to be careful to eat enough alkaline food and to live on a salt-poor diet for at least two days each week. If these two days are faithfully kept, the amount of salt accumulated during the rest of the week will do no harm. Von Noorden, in his pamphlet about Zig Zag Diet, emphasizes the beneficial results in a great many diseases from "changed-diet-days."

Most patients, who are concerned in this problem, are constitutionally bound, children as well as adults, to be subject to colds and sinus infections, and should therefore be made conscious that diet and certain rules in life will be just as important to them as to people who suffer from high blood pressure, kidney and heart diseases.

XXI

THE MANAGEMENT OF THE PATIENT

Much of the success of the dietetic treatment depends upon an intelligent control of the patient. In order to be successful the physician should not only be familiar with the physiological and biochemical side of the diet, but frequently will have to use common sense in discovering the mistakes of the patient, which keep the urine acid, the chlorides high, and prevent success. It goes without saying that the application of the diet does not and cannot exclude surgery entirely from the therapy. Surgery will always have its place in the treatment of sinus diseases, but I feel that dietetic treatment, which so far has been neglected in this field, will do much to bring surgery back within the limits where it belongs.

The following mistakes in the diet seem to be observed most frequently:

1. In spite of having been warned, the patient will still use canned food. One often hears the remark, that this or that has been approved by the Food Committee of the American Medical Association. Any one who understands the principles of the diet will exclude all canned food until time enough has passed to allow the patient to return to a nor-

mal diet for a few days a week. I have seen patients who showed splendid results, receive a setback after attending one banquet.

2. Very frequently one finds that too much bread, starchy desserts and sugar have been eaten. Especially in the beginning of the diet, sugar should be taken only in small amounts and be replaced whenever possible by pure honey. If there is no indication of intestinal disorders, dark rye, graham or pumpernickel bread should be taken exclusively from the beginning.

3. Too much protein may have been taken,— meat, eggs and seafood. Many patients become careless as to the proportions of the food and take considerably more protein than allowed in the diet.

4. The preparation of the food should be carefully controlled. I have seen a great many patients who, though they emphasized the fact that they had faithfully followed instructions, showed by repeated examinations an acid condition. In talking with them I found that they had prepared the food, especially vegetables, in a way which would undoubtedly give them an acid surplus. The attention of the patient must be called again and again to the fact that warming over food will turn it acid.

5. When a strong alkaline urine is found, the controlling physician should be suspicious of alkaline drugs. They are, as a rule, not necessary.

6. Concerning fruit juices—many patients seem to be too lazy to prepare them, and instead of taking a variety of such juices, limit themselves to orange

juice and lemonade. The fruit and vegetable juices should not be diluted with water or sweetened with sugar. They should be taken in large enough amounts to supply the body requirements for water. In ailing and bedridden people, the need for water is limited and all amounts of fluid necessary for the healing should be restricted to fruit and vegetable juices.

7. Some people do not care for the taste of vegetable juices and rather want to restrict these and use other juices which they prefer. I advise them not to do this but to take a variety. If in a sensitive patient, the skin should react with a yellow reddish color, after a large amount of carrot juice has been taken, this juice should be omitted for two or three weeks.

To improve the taste of vegetable juices, they may be mixed with one-fourth of fruit juice. Frequently it is sufficient to add a few drops of lemon juice. Many patients become so used to the juices that they miss them if they are sometimes omitted.

8. The fruit juices should always be taken fresh. Fermentation sets in after a few hours and may influence the action. All juices should be kept cool and put in a glass or porcelain container. Metal and enamel will aid fermentation and alter the taste.

9. If diarrhea is reported the diet schedule must be temporarily changed and fruit and vegetable juices decreased. They may be given with one-half part oatmeal or tapioca, decreasing these as soon as normal digestion is restored.

10. In constipation, which seldom occurs, no laxa-

tive should be used. If necessary an enema will be best using one quart of camomile tea.

11. Some patients think, that when they are put on the diet they must improve at once. If a relapse occurs after two or three weeks one should not become discouraged. I felt, in some cases, that this was due to a focal reaction, similarly as we see it happening in other unspecific and specific treatments. I saw frequently in these patients that the diet later led to a complete cure and resistance against colds.

12. An over-indulgence in alcohol and smoking may have a bad influence and in some cases may make all efforts futile.

13. Patients, who during the diet go about their daily tasks, should be admonished to be sure to eat between meals.

In talking with patients after they have been on the diet for a while, one can hear the most interesting statements from them, of how the diet affected them. A very small group will discontinue the diet because of a lack of appetite for unsalted food, or because of the impossibility of devoting the necessary time to the preparation of the meals. The majority, however, will enthusiastically follow the instructions. Many patients report that, while perspiring profusely before the diet, they did not perspire so much after four or five days of the treatment, some reporting very happily, that the offensive odor had disappeared. A number of these patients suffered from eczema and skin irritations in the axilla, groin or below the breasts. These skin affections, while present for many months, disappeared within a week or two after the diet had been applied. I remember one patient, a woman of 55, who had suffered for years from pruritus of the genitals and anus. She consulted a skin specialist, who advised her to have seven teeth and her tonsils removed, which was done. After six months she was still suffering from the same symptoms. The dermatologist then referred her to me because he was suspicious of her sinuses. In taking the history, I found that together with her other ailments she had suffered for over ten years from frequent colds and hoarseness. The clinical examinations and X-ray of the nose revealed the fact that every sinus was clouded and diseased. However, no free pus could be obtained in washing her sinuses. When she heard this diagnosis, she wanted to submit to a sinus operation at once. But after explaining that one operation would not be sufficient, because all the sinuses were affected, and suggesting the diet, she became very skeptical and consulted some one else. Four weeks later she returned, saying that the other doctor, whom she had consulted, wanted to charge her a fee which she was unable to pay, and so she thought that before assuming such heavy expense she would try the diet. After being on the diet for two weeks, she reported the disappearance of the itching and of the eczema around the genitals, which was evidently due to the high acidity of her urine. Four weeks later an X-ray of her sinuses revealed the fact that they were all clear. I report this history because it seems to me to contain many of the problems with which we are confronted in our daily practice.

Other patients report the loss of their bad breath, and a large per cent felt relieved from rheumatic and neuritic pains. The attending physician should be well aware of these facts, because these concomitant complaints will frequently improve sooner than the condition of the mucous membranes of the nose.

Statements of patients as mentioned above, will therefore be the best indicators for the physician that the diet has been carried out correctly and that good results may be expected.

Most patients will report, if asked, to have urinated a larger amount than usual. This increase in the diuresis depends on the amount of chlorides found in the previous examinations of urine. The higher the chloride content in the urine, the larger the loss of water after salt is restricted. Together with the loss of water we naturally find a loss of weight. Figuring that 1 gm of salt retains 70 gm of water, one can closely foretell how much weight a patient is bound to lose. This loss of weight, however, is a pleasant and welcome event for all those who are overweight. In patients, who are underweight, the loss of weight due to the elimination of water does not amount to very much, and will soon be replaced by fat and proteins.

REFERENCES

ASCHNER, B.: Die Krise der Medizin, Vol. I. Hippokrates Verlag, 1931.

BARBORKA, C. J.: Proceedings of the Staff of the Mayo Clinic, 6: 461 (August 5, 1931)

BALZLI, H.: Kunst and Wissenschaft des Essens, Zürich, 1930. 2 vols.

BERG, R.: Nahrungs-und Genussmittel, 5th Ed. Dresden, 1929.

—— Vitamin, New York, 1923.

—— Alltägliche Wunder, 5th Ed. Dresden.

—— Eiweissbedarf und Mineralstoffwechsel. Dresden, 1931.

BERG, R.-VOGLE, M.: Grundlagen einer richtigen Ernährung, 7th Ed. Dresden, 1930.

BIRCHER-BENNER: Eine neue Ernährungslehre, 4th Ed. Zürich, 1928.

BLATHERWICK, N. R.: The Specific Rôle of Foods in Relation to the Composition of the Urine. Arch. Int. Med., 1914. 14: 409.

CHITTENDEN, R. H.: The Nutrition of Man. New York, 1907.

EKBLAW: Quoted according to McCollum.

EPPINGER, H., and ULLMAN, E. V.: Zur Frage des Kalkstoffwechsels. Wiener Archiv f. Int. Med. 1. Band, 1920.

FALTA: Wien. klin. Woch. 1930, 148.

GERSON, M.: Meine Diet. Ullstein, 1930. Berlin.

GLASSCHEIB, A.: Uber den Einfluss der Ernährung auf

die Rhinitis vasomotoria Monatssch. f. Ohrenheil-
kunde, 62: 2: 1928.

HINDHEDE, M.: Moderne Ernährung. Berlin W. Vobach,
1915.

—— Eine Reform unserer Ernährung. Kopenhagen, 1908.

HUTCHISON, J. W.: On Greenland's Closed Shores. Edin-
borough and London. W. Blackwood, 1930.

JARVIS, D. C.: Upper Respiratory Tract, a Guide to Nutritional Diseases. Ann. of Otol. Rhin. Lar. 39:
584-592. June, 1930.

—— The Red Nasal Septum Syndrome. Ann. of Otol.
Rhin. Lar. XLI: 4. Dec., 1932: 1124.

KROETZ: Münchner med. Woch., 1929, p. 1988.

KUSZINSKI: Quoted by R. Berg.

LUITHLEN, K.: Kationenverhältnis bei verschiedener Ernährung Arch f. exp. Pathol. 68: 209: 1912.

—— Vorlesungen ueber Pharmakolgie der Haut. Berlin,
1921.

McCOLLUM and SIMMON: The Newer Knowledge of Nutrition. Macmillan, 1925.

McCRACKER, H.: God's Frozen Children. Doubleday,
Doran & Co., 1930.

MITTERMAIER, R.: Untersuchungen über die Hydrogen-
ion Concentration an Sekreten und Schleimhäuten,
in besonderen bei chron. Nasennebenhöhlener-
krankungen. Arch. f. Ohren-Nasen usw., 1930.
127: 1.

NOORDEN, VON: Über Zick-Zack Kost. Therapie d.
Gegenwart, 1931. 1.

—— Alte und neuzeitliche Ernärungsfragen Wien-Berlin,
J. Springer, 1931.

NOORDEN-SALOMON: Allgemeine Dietetik. Berlin, 1920.

—— Handbuch der Pathologie d. Stoffwechsels. Berlin,
1908.

OSBORNE, T. B., and MENDEL, L. B.: The Use of Soya

Bean Flour as Food. Journal Biol. Chem., 1918. XXXII, 369.

——Inorganic Elements of Nutrition. Journal Biol. Chem., 1918. XXXIV, 1931.

PEMBERTON, R.: Arthritis and Rheumathoid Conditions, their Nature and Treatment. Philadelphia, 1930.

PLIMMER, R. H. A.: Practical Organic and Biochemistry. London, New York, Longmans, Green & Co., 1915.

ROERICH, G. N.: Trails to Inmost Asia. Oxford Press, 1931.

RUBNER, M.: Alte und neue Irrewege auf dem Gebiete der Volksernährung. Berlin, 1929.

SALKOWSKI, E.: Ueber die Wirkung der Säuren im Organismus. Arch f. exper. Pathol. u Pharm. 1877, VII.

SANSUM, W. D.: The Normal Diet. 3d Ed. C. V. Mosby Co., St. Louis, 1930.

SAUERBRUCH, F.: Wundinfektion, Wundheilung und Entzündung Münchner med. Woch. 1924, 38.

SAUERBRUCH-HERMANNSDORFER-GERSON: Uber Versuche, schwere Formen der Tuberculose durch dietetische Behandlung zu beeinflussen. Münch med. Woch., 1926. 11, 111.

STRAUSS, H.: Zur Frage der Dietbehandlung der Lungentuberkulose Med. Klinik 25, 1383 (Sept. 6), 929.

TOM, CHARLES: Quoted from A. H. McCann: The Science of Keeping Young, New York, George W. Doran & Co., page 367, 1926.

ULLMANN, E. V.: Chronic Sinus Diseases, Their Dietetic Treatment. Northwest Medicine, 31: 240. May, 1932.

——The Principles of a New Diet applied to Patients suffering from Sinus Diseases and Frequent Colds. Clinical Medicine and Surgery, Nov., 1932.

—— Dietetic Treatment of Sinus Diseases. The Laryngoscope, 42: 552, Aug., 1932.

ULLMANN, E. V., and EPPINGER, H.: Zur Frage des Kalkstoffwechsels. Wiener Archiv f. Int. Med. 1. Band, 1920.

URBACH, E.: Skin Diseases and Nutrition. Wilh. Maudrich, Vienna, 1932.

VEIT, E.: Ztschr f. Biol. 1901, III.

WIDAL, F., and JAVAL, A.: La Cure de Dechloruration. Paris, 1913. Librairie Baillière.

WOLFF-EISNER, A.: Kochsalzzufuhr bei Gesunden und Kranken. Med. Welt, 51: 1929.

APPENDIX
By ELSA MEZ

RECIPES AND MENUS

Years of experience with dietary regimes for sick and healthy people alike have taught me that the secret of a correct physiological and psychological approach is not so much in the avoidance or interdiction of certain undesirable though "piquant" foods, but rather in a gradual substitution of even better-tasting dishes of a rational diet.

The suggestions presented in these pages are easy to follow. A keen enjoyment will be found in the challenge to apply the family budget to palatable and healthful eating rather than to drugstore or doctor bills.

These recipes are meant for two persons, unless otherwise stated.

ELSA MEZ.

SOUPS

(For occasional use)

Vegetable Soup. Chop 1 onion, 2 carrots, celery, 1 potato, add parsley, 1 bay leaf, a few grains of nutmeg and boil. Flavor with 1 tablespoon butter and a little thyme.

Potato Soup. 3 potatoes, 1 onion and celery are boiled in water. When done pass through potato dicer, then heat 2 tablespoons butter, and pour soup into butter, add 1 tablespoon lemon juice, 1 tablespoon chopped parsley or chives and some summer savory. Before serving add ⅓ cup of sour cream.

Split Pea Soup. Soak split peas over night (⅔ water to ⅓ peas) and boil the next day. Add 2 more cups of water and boil until peas dissolve into a thick soup. Brown 2 tablespoons of whole wheat bread croutons in 4 tablespoons butter and add to soup, also 1 tablespoon vinegar and 2 tablespoons sour cream.

Lentil Soup. Soak lentils over night. Boil and mash through collander. Brown 1 minced onion in butter, add to soup and flavor with lemon juice and nutmeg.

FISH

These dishes are always for 2 or more persons

Baked Halibut. 2 tablespoons sweet butter are heated in a pan, add ½ sliced onion, some chopped parsley, ⅓ teaspoon allspice, put the piece of fish in it, add half a cup of water and 2 tablespoons vinegar, baste from time to time, until flesh separates from bones. To the sauce add ⅓ cup of sour cream and 1 teaspoon whole wheat flour, sprinkle with freshly chopped parsley.

Any large piece of fish or whole fish can be baked in this manner.

Boiled Salmon (Trout or Barracuda). In 2 cups of water boil parsley, 1 bay leaf, 2 cloves, 2 tablespoons vinegar, 1 slice lemon, some celery and a few peppercorns, ½ sliced onion and the fish. (Let water come to a boil, then simmer until the fish is done.) Serve with Sauce Hollandaise.

Broiled Mackerel. Wipe and dry fish well, make an incision along the bone, and put into it a piece of butter, a pinch of allspice and a few drops of vinegar, broil slowly from ten to 15 minutes or until done, serve with Parsley Sauce.

Fish in Gelatine. Salmon, Bluefish, Flounder or Cod may be used.

In 2 cups of water boil 1 sliced onion, 1 teaspoon chopped parsley, ⅓ teaspoon sage, 2 slices lemon, then add fish and simmer slowly until done. Break the piece of fish into small flakes and put into mold. Dissolve 2 tablespoons Knox Gelatin (still better Battle Creek vegetable gelatine, and stir into the simmering fish water, dissolve gelatine completely and pour over fish flakes in mold. When stiff, serve on lettuce leaves and mayonnaise.

Clams and Oysters. Clams and oysters can be used raw or cooked.

Lobsters, Crabs, Shrimps. Lobsters, Crabs and Shrimps should only be used, when they have been bought alive and boiled in saltless water.

Smelts, Perch, etc. Smelts, perch and other small fish may be fried whole in sweet butter. Do not roll in bread crumbs or flour.

MEAT

(for more than 2 persons)

Meats, dried beans, peas, lentils are restricted in use as indicated in text on account of high protein content.

Broiled Steak. Grease gridiron with butter, broil steak over clear fire, turning every ten seconds, cook from four to five minutes, serve with Maître d'Hôtel butter.

Lamb Chops. Have frying pan hot with butter, put in chops and sear on both sides quickly, then cover and cook slowly until done. Make a sauce with 1 tablespoon whole wheat flour, 1 tablespoon chopped cooked mushrooms, 2 tablespoons of sour cream.

Veal or Pork Roast. Put 3 tablespoons butter in kettle and heat, add one chopped onion and meat and sear on all sides. Add 2 tablespoons water and bake in oven, in covered pan, allowing half an hour to one pound. When half done, add 1 tablespoon each of chopped parsley and chopped celery, ½ teaspoon mustard, 2 tablespoons fresh or dried mushrooms, 1 cup of water and baste often until done. To the sauce add 2 tablespoons cream.

Rabbit and Veal Fricassee. These may be prepared in the same way as Chicken fricassee.

Irish Stew. 2 pounds of lamb stew may be seared slightly in hot butter. Slice 2 onions, 6 carrots, a small cabbage and 3 potatoes and add to the meat. Cover with hot water and boil until done. Add 1 tablespoon parmesan cheese, 1 bay leaf, a few grains paprika and 2 tomatoes and simmer slowly until soup has slightly thickened.

Liver. Sauté ½ sliced onion in butter, add liver and fry lightly on both sides for five minutes. To the sauce add 1 teaspoon of whole wheat flour, 1 teaspoon lemon juice or vinegar, ⅓ cup sour cream and 2 tablespoons water, stir well and pour over liver. Serve immediately.

Braised Sweetbreads. Wash sweetbreads, put in hot butter with fried onions, parsley and a pinch of allspice, cover with water and bake in oven 35 to 40 minutes.

Scalloped Brains. Parboil brains; sprinkle with paprika and lemon juice. Cut in inch pieces, arrange in layers in buttered baking dish, alternating with slices of onions and tomatoes. Cover with butter and grated parmesan cheese and bake 30 to 40 minutes.

POULTRY

Fryers. Heat 2 tablespoons sweet butter in pan, cut up one-half onion and fry with the chicken over the open fire, after 10 minutes add half tomato, 3 tablespoons sour cream, 1 tablespoon wine vinegar, ⅓ cup of water and bake 10 minutes more.

Pigeons. Pigeons may be prepared in the same manner.

Roast Goose. Peel and slice 2 apples, 1 onion, ½ raw potato, to this add ⅓ teaspoon sage, 1 teaspoon parmesan cheese, 1 tablespoon wine vinegar and one beaten egg, and stuff goose with mixture, then sew, and place in buttered pan, bake for one hour, add one cup of water and baste from time to time until tender and brown. When done take superfluous fat off, and add 1 tablespoon whole wheat flour to the gravy, a few grains of cayenne and 1 tablespoon of lemon juice.

Turkey Stuffing No. 1. 1 cup whole wheat crumbs seasoned with sage, thyme and allspice, ½ cup melted butter, 1 beaten egg, 1 apple cut into small pieces, ½ cup of seedless raisins, 1 tomato and hot water to make it quite moist.

Turkey Stuffing No. 2. ½ sliced onion, 1 cup of boiled chestnuts, 1 stalk of celery, some raisins, ½ cup of melted butter, 1 beaten egg, 1 tablespoon wine vinegar, ½ teaspoon poultry seasoning.

Roast Turkey. Stuff turkey, sew and put in pan with hot butter; brown in oven, then add 1½ cups of hot water, baste often and cook until legs separate from body. Take turkey out and make a gravy with 2 tablespoons whole wheat flour, ½ cup of sour cream and 1 tablespoon lemon juice and more water if needed.

Roast Chicken. Roast chicken may be prepared in the same way as Roast Turkey.

Chicken Fricassee. Cut chicken at the joints into pieces. Put in kettle with butter, let brown lightly, add 2 tablespoons whole wheat flour and let brown, then cover chicken with boiling water. Season with 2 slices of lemon, ⅓ teaspoon poultry seasoning, 2 cloves, a few grains of nutmeg, 1 bay leaf. Simmer until tender, stir in one beaten egg and half a cup of sour cream or 1 tablespoon of parmesan cheese. Mushrooms may be added, too.

EGG DISHES

Cheese Soufflé. Beat 4 egg-whites very stiff, to this add the 4 egg-yolks beaten well, 3 tablespoons grated parmesan cheese, a few grains of paprika, 1 teaspoon whole wheat flour dissolved in ½ cup of cold milk, beat together lightly, turn into buttered baking dish, and bake 20 minutes, serve immediately.

Spinach Omelette à la Mez. Boil spinach, chop fine and add 1 tablespoon butter. Mix ½ cup of whole wheat flour with 2 egg-yolks, ¾ cup of milk, beat egg-whites and fold in lightly. Melt 1 teaspoon butter in frying pan and bake very thin omelettes. Put one after the other into buttered baking dish, fill each one with a large tablespoon spinach, roll up, sprinkle with parmesan cheese and bake 10 minutes in oven.

Russian Eggs. Boil eggs hard, peel and cut into halves. Take out egg-yolk, mash with a fork and add ½ finely chopped onion, 1 tablespoon chopped parsley, 1 teaspoon unsalted mustard, 1 large tablespoon mayonnaise, a little paprika, mix well and refill the halves of the boiled egg-whites and serve on nest of watercress.

Eggs in Mustard Sauce. Poach eggs; prepare a mustard sauce; melt 1 tablespoon butter, dissolve 1 tablespoon whole wheat flour in ¾ cup of water and add to butter, stir until it thickens. Put in 1 large teaspoon of unsalted mustard, 1 teaspoon vinegar, 1 teaspoon chopped chives, stir well and pour over poached eggs.

Scrambled Eggs. Beat two whole eggs, add ½ cup of sour or sweet cream and 1 teaspoon parmesan cheese, heat butter in frying pan and scramble lightly.

Omelettes. Mix together 1 cup of whole wheat flour, 2 beaten egg-yolks, ¾ cup of milk, and fold in beaten egg-whites. Heat butter in frying pan, put in 2 tablespoons of dough, spread and bake quickly, put flat into buttered baking dish, fill with 1 tablespoon of marmalade, roll up omelette, sprinkle with brown sugar and cinnamon and bake for five minutes in oven.

Filled Omelettes. Prepare as above, but instead of marmalade, fill with cauliflower or mushrooms, sprinkle with parmesan cheese and bake.

Scrambled Eggs with Tomatoes. Scramble eggs as above, add sliced boiled onion and tomatoes.

VEGETABLES

Vegetables may be cooked in three different ways, *always without salt*. First, they may be steamed in water. Not less than three tablespoons of water and not more than one cup (according to quantity of vegetables) should be added. To avoid burning they are simmered after they have come to a boil. It usually requires not more than half an hour for any kind of vegetable to cook, provided it is cooked in a tightly covered container.

Second, they may be sautéed. Heat 2 tablespoons of olive oil or butter in a kettle, and put in the cleaned and washed vegetable, cover tightly, but turn frequently to avoid scorching. Third, vegetables may be baked in the oven in buttered baking dishes, which should also be covered with a closs-fitting lid; before serving, the cover may be removed to brown top layer.

Vegetable Soufflé. Slice 2 raw potatoes, two tomatoes and squash. Brown one sliced onion. Butter baking dish and put in layers of each. On top add the onion, a few slices of butter, $\frac{1}{3}$ cup of water with 1 tablespoon vinegar, sprinkle with grated parmesan cheese, and bake for half an hour in hot oven.

Spinach Soufflé. Wash and steam spinach (no water added), grind through food chopper. Soak 1 slice of whole wheat bread in water, squeeze out and add to the spinach, also half a cup of sour cream, three egg-yolks, 1 tablespoonful lemon juice; beat egg-whites and fold in. Put this mixture into buttered baking dish, sprinkle with parmesan cheese, and bake for 30 minutes in hot oven. Serve with tomato sauce.

Cauliflower au Gratin. Boil cauliflower; when cooked, put into buttered baking dish. Make sauce with the leftover water (about $\frac{1}{2}$ cup). To 2 tablespoons of cold water add 1 tablespoon whole wheat flour, pour this into the broth and let thicken, add 2 tablespoons butter, 1 tablespoon wine vinegar or lemon and at last stir in one egg-yolk. Pour over cauliflower, sprinkle with 1 tablespoon grated parmesan cheese and brown lightly in oven.

Stuffed Tomatoes. Cut off a slice from top of tomato, scoop out pulp and mix with equal quantities of cooked brown rice and minced brown onion; season with paprika and chopped parsley. Refill tomatoes, cover with the tops, sprinkle with parmesan cheese and bake for 20 minutes.

Onions. Peel onions and boil in a little water, add one tablespoon chopped parsley, 2 tablespoons of butter and 1 tablespoon sour cream and 1 tablespoon vinegar (instead of vinegar Curtasal can be used).

String Beans. Remove the strings and slice at an angle into thin slices, add one-half sliced onion and cook. For seasoning add 2 tablespoons wine vinegar, chopped parsley and nutmeg.

French Spinach. Wash spinach thoroughly, boil without water slowly for 5 minutes, put through grinder, put back in kettle to heat, add 3 tablespoons of sweet cream, a few drops of lemon juice, 1 tablespoon sweet butter, and if too watery, add one teaspoon whole wheat flour to thicken.

Green Peas. Shell, boil and season with lemon juice, butter, parsley and a dash of marjoram.

Eggplant. Peel and cut into thin slices. Heat two tablespoons butter and 2 tablespoons olive oil and sauté them in this until lightly browned. Sprinkle with nutmeg and lemon juice or vinegar. While frying cut up some chives and fry with it.

Tomatoes. Boil tomatoes and one large onion, a stalk of small celery sliced, 1 bayleaf and a little sage. Season with sour cream and butter.

Squash. Cut squash into pieces, boil 10 minutes, add 2 tablespoons sweet butter, a teaspoon lemon juice and sour cream.

Cooked Lettuce. Pick over and wash each leaf, break into smaller pieces. Simmer in 2 tablespoons water for 10 minutes, and add one teaspoon parsley or chives, a large piece butter and a few drops of lemon juice.

Sauerkraut. Wash out three times to remove salt, boil with ½ cup water until soft, add one bayleaf and a few peppercorns, when done prepare with butter, 1 apple and one potato can be boiled with it, if desired.

Brussels Sprouts. Wash well and pick off yellow leaves, boil in a little water, add butter and sour cream.

Kohlrabi. Wash kohlrabi, boil and peel when tender by pulling the tough skin off. Slice and serve in white sauce.

Filled Kohlrabi. Boil kohlrabi as above, cut a slice off the top, scoop out with a spoon, add to this a mixture of chopped parsley, sour cream, chopped browned onions, butter and nutmeg, refill, cover with tops, put in buttered baking dish, sprinkle with parmesan cheese and bake for 20 minutes.

Filled Cabbage Leaves. Peel off the large leaves of a cabbage, boil until half done and fill. Filling: 1 slice of soaked whole wheat bread, 1 tomato cut into small pieces, 1 chopped onion, chopped sage, 1 beaten egg, 1 tablespoon vinegar, mix this well, put 1 large spoonful into the cabbage leaf, roll up, and put the rolls closely together in a buttered baking dish, add a little water and butter. Bake for 20 minutes or until nicely browned.

Peas and Carrots. Wash and scrub carrots well, cut into thin slices, add peas and boil. For seasoning add large piece of butter, 1 tablespoon vinegar, 1 teaspoon brown sugar, 1 tablespoon chopped parsley.

Eggplant and String Beans. Brown one sliced onion in butter, peel and slice one eggplant, put into kettle with onion, add 3 tablespoons of water and parboil. To this can be added leftover string beans or carrots; for seasoning use 1 tablespoon horseradish, chopped parsley, 1 tablespoon vinegar, butter and nutmeg and finish cooking.

Salsify. Wash and scrub salsify well, boil and peel, and cut into long slices and serve with white sauce.

Salsify Souffié à la Ullmann. Prepare salsify as before, put into buttered baking dish, add one egg-yolk to white sauce, pour over salsify and sprinkle with parmesan cheese, bake for 10 minutes.

Sautéed Bananas. Peel bananas and cut into half lengthwise. Sprinkle with a few drops of lemon juice and dust lightly with whole wheat flour. Heat 1 tablespoon olive oil and 1

tablespoon butter and sauté bananas until brown, add 1 teaspoon brown sugar and serve.

Asparagus. Peel asparagus by cutting the hard skin off up to
the tender green part. Boil for 20 to 30 minutes. With the
leftover water make the following sauce: To ½ cup of
asparagus water add 2 tablespoons lemon juice, 2 tablespoons
butter, 1 teaspoon brown sugar, and 1½ tablespoons whole
wheat flour, stir over fire until it thickens, then add one
beaten egg-yolk, stir well, fold in beaten egg-white, and pour
over asparagus.

POTATOES

Potatoes should always be boiled with the skin

Parsley Potatoes. Wash and boil potatoes, peel, cut into
squares, add one large tablespoon butter and 1 tablespoon
chopped parsley.

Mashed Potatoes. Wash, boil and peel potatoes, mash, add
milk, butter and nutmeg and beat until light.

Raw Potatoes with Apples. Wash and scrub potatoes with a
brush, then slice on fine slicer. Peel and slice 1 or 2 apples
and one onion. Heat a tablespoon of butter in frying pan
and place potatoes, apples and onion in it. Fry golden
brown, add a piece of butter from time to time and a little
paprika (Curtasal if desired).

Baked Potatoes. Wash and clean well, dry and rub with olive
oil, bake in hot oven about 40 minutes or until soft, break
the skin to let the steam escape. Serve with sweet butter.

Potato Souffle. Scrub and bake potatoes, when done cut
lengthwise into halves, and scoop out with spoon. Mash this,
add 1 large tablespoon of butter, 1 tablespoon hot milk, a
few grains of nutmeg, 1 tablespoon grated parmesan cheese,
folding in 2 beaten egg-whites. Fill the skins with this mixture and bake in oven for 15 minutes.

Potato Balls. Mash hot potatoes, add chopped parsley and
onion, 1 tablespoon melted butter, 1 beaten egg, ⅓ teaspoon
nutmeg, roll in a little whole wheat flour and bake in hot
butter to a golden brown.

Sautéed Potatoes with Onions. Peel cold boiled potatoes, also one large onion. Put in buttered pan and bake until crisp and brown, add some more butter if needed, season with 1 teaspoon lemon juice and nutmeg.

Sautéed Sweet Potatoes. Peel and slice cold sweet potatoes, heat 1 tablespoon olive oil and 1 tablespoon butter in frying pan, add potatoes and bake nicely brown, add 1 teaspoon brown sugar and a dash of cinnamon.

Sweet Potatoes. Wash potatoes, oil the skin and bake for 45 minutes or until soft.

Caraway seed Potatoes. Wash potatoes, cut in halves, put into pie plate and spread butter over them, sprinkle with caraway seed and bake for 30 minutes or until done.

Creamed Potatoes. Boil potatoes with the skin, then peel and cut into slices. Put into kettle, add ½ a cup of sweet cream, chopped parsley or chives, nutmeg, 2 tablespoons butter and 1 tablespoon vinegar.

Baked Potato Dish. Heat 3 tablespoons butter, brown one sliced onion, 3 carrots, 1 stalk of chopped celery, add 3 washed, scraped and sliced potatoes, cover with ⅔ water and boil slowly, when nearly done add nutmeg, chopped chives, 1 tablespoon wine vinegar, sprinkle with 1 tablespoon grated parmesan cheese and bake for 10 minutes in oven.

Potato Pancakes. 3 large potatoes are washed, scraped and then grated on coarse grater. Put into strainer and let some of the water drain off. To potato pulp add 2 beaten eggs, nutmeg and one tablespoon whole wheat flour, 1 teaspoon vinegar (or Curtasal for seasoning instead). Heat 2 tablespoons olive oil and 1 tablespoon butter together, put 1 tablespoon of potato into it, spread to thin round cake and bake until brown. Serve with apple sauce.

Mashed Potatoes au Gratin. Prepare mashed potatoes without milk, but 2 egg-yolks, and fold in 2 beaten egg-whites, put into buttered baking dish, sprinkle with 1 tablespoon grated parmesan cheese, put a few small pieces of butter on top and bake for 15 to 20 minutes.

RICE

Only unpolished brown rice should be used

Boiled Rice. Wash rice well and boil ⅓ rice in ⅔ water. Let come to boil, then cover and simmer for 30 minutes.

Tomato Rice. Slice 2 large peeled tomatoes and one onion and add to parboiled rice. Before serving pour 4 tablespoons browned butter over it.

Risotto. Boil rice; beat two whole eggs and add 2 tablespoons of sweet butter and 3 tablespoons grated parmesan cheese, pour rice into this mixture, beat well and serve in covered dish.

Baked Rice. Boil rice, then add 2 egg-yolks, 2 tablespoons parmesan cheese, ½ cup of milk, nutmeg, fold in egg-whites, pour into buttered baking dish and bake lightly brown.

Rice Balls. To cold boiled rice add 1 beaten egg, ½ chopped and browned onion, 1 tablespoon cottage cheese, form little balls and bake in 1 tablespoon butter and 2 tablespoons olive oil nicely brown.

SALADS

Salad Dressings

Mayonnaise Dressing No. 1. Beat one whole egg with a few drops of lemon juice and half a teaspoon brown sugar, then add pure olive oil, drop by drop, continuously beating it until mixture begins to thicken; continue until it reaches desired thickness. Add 1 tablespoon vinegar and a few grains of paprika. Keep in a cool place.

Dressing No. 2. Rub mixing bowl with onion or garlic; mix a few grains of paprika with olive oil and vinegar and stir well.

Sour Cream Dressing No. 3. Whip half cup of sour cream, add 1 teaspoon brown sugar and the juice of half a lemon and beat well.

Mustard Dressing No. 4. 2 hard-boiled egg-yolks, a finely minced onion and 1 teaspoon unsalted mustard are mixed with half a cup of sour cream and the juice of half a lemon; some chopped parsley may be added.

Raw Salads

Lettuce. Separate lettuce leaves, wash and drain, put in salad bowl and serve with dressing No. 2. Mix well.

Lettuce with Sour Cream. Separate lettuce leaves, wash and drain, put in a large mixing bowl, and prepare with half a cup of sour cream, with 1 tablespoon vinegar, and 1 teaspoon brown sugar.

Endive Salad. Wash and drain leaves, marinate with dressing No. 2, and sprinkle with chopped chives.

Watercress Salad. Remove leaves from stems, wash and drain, chop one peeled apple into little squares, add to watercress and serve with dressing No. 1 or 2.

Tomato and Lettuce. Arrange peeled and sliced tomatoes on a nest of shredded lettuce, serve with dressing No. 1 to which chopped onion or chives are added.

Stuffed Tomatoes No. 1. Remove the skin from tomatoes, scoop out the inside and to the pulp add chopped celery, nuts and apples, mix with dressing No. 1, refill shells. Serve on watercress.

Stuffed Tomatoes No. 2. Fill tomato shell with minced chicken and celery, add dressing No. 1.

Stuffed Tomatoes No. 3. Refill tomato shells with equal parts of chopped eggs, tomato-pulp, chopped celery, parsley, and marinate with dressing No. 3.

Pineapple Salad. Peel and slice pineapple, serve with cottage cheese, sprinkle chopped nuts over it.

Cucumber Salad. Peel and slice one cucumber on fine slicer, the thinner the better, add dressing No. 2 and garnish with chopped parsley.

Grated Carrots. Wash and clean carrots, grate or put through meat grinder, serve on lettuce leaves with dressing No. 1.

Red Cabbage Salad. Shave cabbage very fine; heat half a cup of wine vinegar, add two teaspoons brown sugar, half a teaspoon mustard, pour over cabbage and mix well.

Apple Salad. Peel and slice apples, chop nuts and celery, add raisins and serve on lettuce leaves, with dressing No. 3.

Radish Salad. Wash and grate radishes, add dressing No. 2, and serve on nest of watercress.

Cooked Salads

Vegetable Salad. Slice boiled carrots, add boiled beans and mix with dressing No. 2, sprinkle with chopped parsley and ⅓ minced onion and serve on lettuce leaves.

Beet Salad. Wash and boil red beets, peel and slice very fine. Mince half an onion, to this add 2 tablespoons vinegar, 2 teaspoons brown sugar and mix well.

Bean Salad. Boil string beans and serve with dressing No. 2 to which chopped parsley and chives have been added.

Celery Root Salad. Wash and scrub celery root well, boil until tender, cut off the brown skin and slice very fine, prepare with dressing No. 2, and serve on nest of endive.

Parsnip Salad. Wash, boil and peel parsnips, cut into slices and add dressing No. 2, sprinkle with chopped chives.

Salsify Salad. May be prepared in the same way.

Chicken Salad. Cut boiled chicken meat (or leftover) into small pieces, add ½ chopped onion, ½ stalk of minced celery, serve with dressing No. 1 on lettuce leaves.

Fish Salad. Boil fish in 1 cup of water to which has been added 1 bayleaf, 2 slices of lemon, a few slices of onion, ¼ teaspoon nutmeg and 2 tablespoons cider vinegar. When fish is tender, break into small flakes, and mix with ½ minced onion and celery. Serve on lettuce leaves with dressing No. 1.

Cauliflower Salad. Boil cauliflower, break into small pieces, serve on nest of watercress with dressing No. 1.

Potato Salad. Boil and peel potatoes, slice fine while still warm, add ½ mince onion, chopped parsley and mix with 2 tablespoons pure olive oil, 2 tablespoons vinegar, ½ teaspoon brown sugar, a few grains of nuetmeg and 1 tablespoon warm water. Stir lightly so as not to break up potatoes. To be served warm.

Boiled Egg Salad. Boil eggs hard, cut into squares, place on sliced tomatoes, and serve on shredded lettuce with dressing No. 4.

Artichoke Salad. Boil artichokes, let cool and serve on lettuce leaves with dressing No. 1.

SAUCES

Sauce Hollandaise. Cream half a cup of sweet butter, add 3 egg-yolks, one at a time, beat well, add 2 tablespoons wine vinegar, half teaspoon brown sugar and a pinch of cayenne; before serving add ½ cup of boiling water, stir well and place in double boiler, stir rapidly until it thickens like custard.

Horseradish Sauce No. 1. Grate fresh horseradish and add ½ cup of sour cream and 2 tablespoons vinegar, 1 teaspoon brown sugar.

Horseradish Sauce No. 2. Grate fresh horseradish, whip sweet cream, 1 tablespoon lemon juice and mix.

Horseradish Sauce No. 3. Melt 1 tablespoon butter, add 1 tablespoon whole wheat flour and water, 2 tablespoons vinegar, 1 teaspoon brown sugar and make a thick white sauce; to this add the grated horseradish and let simmer for 10 minutes.

Parsley Sauce. Heat 3 tablespoons butter, thicken with 1 tablespoon whole wheat flour. Add water and 2 tablespoons chopped parsley, 1 tablespoon wine vinegar, a little brown sugar and nutmeg.

Cold Parsley Sauce. Chop parsley very fine, add 2 tablespoons Italian olive oil, 1 egg-yolk, 1 tablespoon vinegar, a little pepper, ½ teaspoon unsalted mustard, 2 tablespoons sour cream and beat well until it thickens.

Celery Sauce. Cook 2 stalks of celery in 1 cup of water until tender, mash through colander; melt 2 tablespoons butter, add 1 tablespoon whole wheat flour to thicken and stir well, then add 1 tablespoon lemon juice and ½ teaspoon honey and celery.

Tomato Sauce. Boil one pound of tomatoes in 1 cup of water, rub through a strainer; heat 2 tablespoons butter, stir in 2 tablespoons whole wheat flour, add strained tomato juice gradually and season with paprika, vinegar and brown sugar.

Hot Tartar Sauce. 1 tablespoon vinegar, 1 teaspoon lemon juice; mix in a small bowl and heat over hot water, brown ⅓ cup of butter and strain into mixture.

Maître d'Hôtel Butter. ⅓ cup sweet butter, 1 tablespoon

chopped parsley, 1 tablespoon lemon juice, 1 teaspoon vinegar, a little paprika and ½ teaspoon brown sugar. Rub butter to cream and add ingredients.

Mustard Sauce. Dissolve 1½ tablespoon whole wheat flour in 1 cup of water, boil until it thickens, add 1 tablespoon butter, ½ teaspoon brown sugar, 1 tablespoon cider vinegar and 1 tablespoon French mustard, stir well and boil for a few minutes.

Mushoom Sauce. Boil fresh mushrooms (or dried) in 1 cup of water, when cooked thicken with whole wheat flour, add butter, lemon juice, chopped parsley and nutmeg to taste.

Hot Sour Cream Sauce. Make a thick whole wheat flour sauce; before serving, add ½ cup sour cream, 1 teaspoon brown sugar, 1 tablespoon vinegar and stir well.

Onion Sauce. Sauté minced onion in butter, add flour to thicken, 1 tablespoon sweet cream and 1 tablespoon grated parmesan cheese; keep hot but do not boil any more.

Asparagus Sauce. Take 1 cup of the water in which asparagus has been boiled, thicken with 1 to 2 tablespoons whole wheat flour, add 3 tablespoons butter, 1 tablespoon lemon juice or vinegar, beat one egg-yolk into mixture, 1 teapsoon brown sugar, beat egg-white and fold in before serving.

Bechamel Sauce. In two tablespoons butter, sauté cut up celery, green onions (cut green part in inch length) one sliced white onion, add 2 tablespoons whole wheat flour and boil, add ½ cup sour cream, flavor with lemon juice and nutmeg and rub through a colander.

White Sauce. Heat 2 tablespoons sweet butter, stir 1 to 2 tablespoons whole wheat flour into it and add gradually 1 cup of water (or half water and milk). Let thicken and flavor with 1 tablespoon vinegar and 1 teaspoon brown sugar.

BREADS

Whole Wheat Bread. In 4 cups of lukewarm water dissolve 1 Fleischmann's yeastcake and 2 tablespoons brown sugar, 1 tablespoon butter (and 1 teaspoon Curtasal, if desired). Stir 3 cups of whole wheat flour into it, then cover with cloth and let stand in warm place until dough has doubled in volume. Usually this takes 45 minutes to one hour. Stir in two more cups of flour, then take out of bowl, put on floured board and knead for 5 to 8 minutes; if mixture sticks to hands, add more flour. Butter baking pan and put in loaf, but fill pan only half full, because the second rising will double the volume again. When it has doubled, put in oven and bake 35 to 45 minutes. Instead of a whole loaf, small rolls may be formed and baked in 15 minutes. In place of 5 cups of whole wheat flour, 3 cups of whole wheat flour and 2 cups of soy bean flour may be used.

Rye and Graham Bread. Prepare as above, but use whole rye flour (100% whole rye flour) and graham flour; bake 45 to 55 minutes.

BREAKFAST CEREALS

Apple-oatmeal. 2 tablespoons steel-cut oatmeal are soaked overnight in 4 tablespoons water. Shortly before breakfast add 1 tablespoon milk or cream, sweeten with 2 teaspoons honey, add the juice of ⅓ lemon, stir well while boiling. Grate two or three unpeeled apples into this mixture. If desired add 1 tablespoon grated walnuts and serve with cream.

Oatmeal. 2 tablespoons Scotch oatmeal are soaked in 5 tablespoons water. In the morning boil oatmeal for 15 minutes, add 2 tablespoons of raisins and serve with honey and cream.

Whole Cornmeal Mush (undegerminated cornmeal). Pour ½ cup of cornmeal into 1 cup of boiling water, stir well; before serving, add 1 tablespoon grated almonds or hazelnuts. Serve with honey and cream.

DESSERTS

Hazelnut Drops or Filberts. Beat 4 egg-whites, add 1 teaspoon lemon juice, ¾ cup of brown sugar and beat well until sugar is dissolved, mix 1 to 1½ cups of grated hazelnuts into it, grease pie plates well, drop 1 teaspoonful at a time, rather far apart, and bake quickly in a hot oven. Burns easily.

Chocolate Drops. Prepare as above, but use 1 cup of brown sugar and 1 to 1½ tablespoons cocoa with it. Bake in the same manner.

Almond Drops. Instead of hazelnuts use grated almonds and prepare the same way.

Almond Cookies. 1 cup whole wheat flour, ½ cup butter, ¾ cup brown sugar, 1 tablespoon lemon juice, 2 eggs; knead together, roll out thin, and cut into slices or squares, bake lightly brown in a quick oven.

Strawberry Shortcake. Warm 1 cup of butter and rub creamy, add ¾ cup of brown sugar and beat until dissolved, stir 2 egg-yolks into it, and alternately mix 2 cups of whole wheat flour and ½ cup of milk into this, then fold in stiffly beaten egg-whites and turn into buttered pan or into muffin pan, bake until dry and brown, test with straw or match. Remove from pan as soon as possible. Cut into thin slices and serve with strawberries and whipped cream.

Apple Pie. 1 cup whole wheat flour, ⅓ cup brown sugar, ½ cup butter, 1 to 2 tablespoons water, mix and knead lightly, roll to fit pie plate; make the edge of the crust quite high, so that the fruit juice will not run out. Slice apples in long thin slices and fill crust, piling high in the middle. Bake until apples are soft and crust slightly browned, sprinkle 1 tablespoon brown sugar over it, some cinnamon and a few drops of lemon juice, return to oven for five minutes, then take out of the tin.

Apricot Pie. Use same crust as above. Remove stones from apricots and fill crust.

Raspberry Pie. Same pie crust filled with raspberries.

Cheese Pie. Same pie crust as above. For filling take 3 tablespoons unsalted cottage cheese, beat well with ½ cup of brown sugar, ½ teaspoon cinnamon, 1 tablespoon lemon juice, rind of one grated lemon, 2 tablespoons melted butter, ½ cup of milk, 3 eggs, beat together until smooth; put into pie crust and bake until the mixture thickens like custard. (2 tablespoons seedless raisins may be added to filling.)

Whole Wheat Cookies à la Mez. 1 cup brown sugar, 1½ cups whole wheat flour, 1 cup of sweet butter, grated lemon rind, 2 tablespoons water. Mix to a dough, roll out thin and cut into rounds or squares, bake quickly to a light brown.

Whole Wheat Raisin Cake. Take 1 cup of butter and rub until creamy, add 1 cup of brown sugar and beat again, beat 3 egg-yolks into this, then 1 cup of whole wheat flour and ½ cup of milk, another cup of whole wheat flour and ¾ cup of raisins mixed with ¼ cup of flour, beat egg-whites and fold in, flavor with grated lemon rind and 1 teaspoon of lemon juice, put into buttered pan and bake in hot oven for 40 minutes, or until a match or straw inserted in the center comes out clean.

Rice Soufflé. Parboil rice, then mix with 2 cups of milk, 3 egg-yolks, brown sugar to taste, ½ cup of raisins and ½ cup chopped dates, fold in beaten egg-white, and bake for 20 minutes in buttered baking dish.

Apple Rice with Whipped Cream. Parboil rice and add milk, 3 tablespoons honey and 2 egg-yolks. Fold in egg-whites. Butter baking dish and put in one layer of rice, add a layer of sliced apples, follow with rice and another layer of apples; sprinkle with cinnamon and add a few slices of butter. Bake for 20 to 30 minutes and serve with whipped cream.

Custard. Beat 3 whole eggs with ⅓ cup of brown sugar and 2 cups of milk. Boil in double boiler until thick.

Caramel Custard. To plain custard add 1 to 2 tablespoons caramel.

Prune Whip. Boil dried prunes, remove stones and mash through colander. Add 1 tablespoon lemon juice, grated lemon rind and 3 beaten egg-whites. Turn into buttered baking dish and bake 15 to 20 minutes. Serve with whipped cream.

Raspberry Foam. Strain 1 box of raspberries through cheese-cloth or fine sieve, add ⅓ cup brown sugar, and ½ pint of whipped cream, mix lightly and chill.

Chestnut Creme. Peel chestnuts, put in hot water and peel off inner skin; then boil slowly in water until tender; mash and add 2 tablespoons brown sugar, 1 tablespoon lemon juice, 2 beaten egg-whites, mix and serve with whipped cream.

Baked Apples. Core apples, arrange in baking dish, fill cavities with honey and lemon juice and bake until apples are tender, adding a teaspoon of butter before taking from oven. Serve with cream.

Strawberry Bavarian Cream. Soak 2 teaspoons gelatine (Battle Creek vegetable gelatine) in cold water, dissolve in boiling water, add strawberries which have been cut into halves and sweetened with brown sugar, whip half pint of cream, and stir together lightly. Pour mixture into mold, chill, garnish with strawberries, and serve.

Apple Soufflé. Steam 3 quartered apples, add 1 tablespoon butter, 2 tablespoons honey, lemon juice and 3 beaten egg-yolks, then fold in the beaten egg-whites, turn into buttered pudding dish and bake for 25 minutes, or until nicely browned. Serve with whipped cream.

ICE CREAMS

Raspberry Ice Cream. Mash berries through fine sieve or squeeze through cheesecloth. To the juice add brown sugar (3 cups of juice, 1 cup of sugar), beat ½ pint of whipping cream and mix with the juice and sugar. Turn into freezer or refrigerator trays and freeze.

Strawberry Ice Cream. Clean and mash one box of strawberries, add half cup of brown sugar, beat and add ½ pint of whipping cream, put mixture into freezer and freeze.

Vanilla Ice Cream. Heat one quart of milk in double boiler, add ¾ cup brown sugar and vanilla (from vanilla beans rather than extract); when milk begins to boil thicken with 1 teaspoon of corn-starch (dissolved in cold water). Beat 3 egg-yolks and stir into milk quickly, and continue stirring until mixture thickens. Then let cool while beating it, otherwise it may curdle. When cold fold in the beaten egg-whites and turn into freezer.

Burned Filbert Ice Cream. To vanilla mixture add 4 tablespoons toasted filberts: To toast filberts: Cut the nuts very fine, heat one teaspoon of butter in frying pan and toast filberts lightly brown.

Caramel Ice Cream. Prepare vanilla ice cream and add caramel. Take one tablespoon of brown sugar and melt to a chocolate brown, add 1 or 2 tablespoons of water to this, boil for a few seconds, then add 2 or 3 tablespoons of this to ice cream, stir and turn into freezer and freeze.

To vanilla ice cream as a foundation may be added: sliced peaches or pineapple.

For mocca ice cream add 1 cup of strong coffee to 2 parts of ice cream.

Apricot Sherbet. Boil apricots (in ⅓ water), add brown sugar to taste, when cold fold in 3 stiffly beaten egg-whites, mix and freeze.

Fruit Ice Cream. Slice peaches and bananas, sugar to taste with brown sugar, add 1 teaspoon lemon juice, whip ½ pint of cream and mix with fruit. Freeze solid without stirring.

Chocolate Ice Cream. Heat 1 quart of milk in double boiler with 2 tablespoons cocoa and ¾ cup brown sugar, mix 1 teaspoon corn-starch, or whole wheat flour with 2 beaten egg-yolks and stir into milk, beat well until it begins to thicken. Cool and fold in the beaten egg-whites, beat ½ pint of whipping cream and put half of it into the ice cream mixture, then freeze, and put the rest of the whipping cream on ice cream when serving.

MENUS *

Bread should not be eaten with meals, unless potatoes or rice are omitted

LUNCH

Boiled salmon with mustard sauce, baked potato, tomato salad, baked apple with cream.

String beans with eggplant, sweet potatoes, radish salad, apple pie and fresh fruit.

Omelettes, cauliflower au gratin, tomatoes stuffed with chicken, strawberries and cream, and cookies.

Veal chops and rice in casserole, cold slaw, Dressing No. 3, raspberry foam.

French spinach with poached egg, cucumber salad, apricot tarts with whipped cream.

Eggplant, parsley sauce, caraway seed, potatoes, lettuce, dressing No. 1, apple pie.

DINNER

Artichokes, with sauce Hollandaise, vegetable salad, chocolate ice cream, hazelnut drops.

Lamb chops, onions, rice, watercress salad, fruit gelatin with whipped cream.

Baked barracuda, with parsley sauce, potato soufflé, lettuce salad, prune whip with whipped cream.

Fresh lima beans, grated carrots on lettuce, stuffed tomatoes, and apple pie.

Boiled fish, baked potato, swiss chard, tomato salad and apple soufflé.

Spinach soufflé with tomato sauce, baked potato, beet salad, strawberry bavarian cream.

* These menus are so arranged, that the luncheon menu on the left balances the dinner menu placed directly opposite on the right.

LUNCH

Fish salad, dressing No. 1, cooked lettuce, parsley, potatoes, fresh fruit.

Eggs in mustard sauce, stuffed tomato salad, 1 slice whole rye bread with butter, dates, raisins, raw apple.

Broiled mackerel with Hollandaise sauce, tomato-lettuce salad, mashed potatoes, fresh fruit.

Artichoke with Dressing No. 1, whole wheat bread, cottage cheese, butter, apple rice with whipped cream.

Vegetable salad, stuffed tomatoes on lettuce, caramel custard and cookies.

Poached eggs, mustard sauce, lettuce with dressing No. 3, rice balls, fresh fruit.

Mushrooms, mashed potatoes, red cabbage salad, fresh raspberries with whipped cream.

Glass of milk, whole rye bread, cottage cheese, stuffed tomatoes (raw) melon in season.

DINNER

Filled kohlrabi, mushroom sauce, brown rice, endive salad, apple soufflé, whipped cream.

Carrots with parsley sauce, celery root salad, bananas sautéed.

Salsify à la Ullmann, with hot sour cream sauce, sautéed sweet potatoes, watercress salad, raspberry ice cream.

Irish stew, radish salad, strawberry bavarian cream, hazelnut drops, fresh fruit.

Steak, Maître d'hôtel butter, spinach, baked potato, sliced tomatoes, raspberry ice cream.

Potato pancakes, carrots, apple sauce, and lettuce salad, vanilla ice cream, almond cookies.

Scalloped brains, boiled potatoes, salsify, cucumber salad, chestnut cream and fresh fruit.

Mashed potatoes, sauerkraut, endive salad, fruit gelatin with whipped cream.

LUNCH

Kohlrabi, cooked lettuce, fried sweet potatoes, cheese pie, fresh fruit.

Spinach omelettes, cucumber salad, strawberry shortcake with whipped cream, fresh fruit.

Small fryer, baked sweet potatoes, French spinach, beet salad, raspberry ice cream.

Risotto, squash, tomato soufflé, peaches with cream, whole wheat cake.

Whole wheat lettuce sandwiches, boiled egg salad, buttermilk, fresh fruit.

DINNER

Vegetable soup, hot artichokes with drawn butter, rice soufflé with stewed fruit.

Broiled mackerel, horseradish sauce No. 1, potato balls, salsify, fruit, bananas, nuts, dates.

Sweet corn, boiled onion, bean salad, lettuce with sour cream dressing, caramel custard, almond cookies.

Liver, spinach, sweet potatoes, cranberries, apricot sherbet.

Turnips, white sauce, sautéed potatoes with apples, pineapple salad, apple soufflé with whipped cream.

GENERAL INDEX

INDEX FOR RECIPES